VESTIBULAR MIGRAINE DIET COOKBOOK

"Cooking For Holistic Health And Relief"

Anita F. MS RDN McCluskey

Copyright © 2024 by Anita F. MS, RDN.McCluskey

All rights reserved. No part of this publication may be reproduced, distributed, or transmitted in any form or by any means, including photocopying, recording, or other electronic or mechanical methods, without the prior written permission of the publisher, except in the case of brief quotations embodied in critical reviews and certain other noncommercial uses permitted by copyright law.

Legal notice: This book is protected by copyright law and is intended for personal use only. Without explicit permission from the publisher or author, you are prohibited from altering, distributing, selling, quoting, or paraphrasing any portion of the book's content.

"Disclaimer:

The recipes and information provided in this "Vestibular Migraine Diet Cookbook" are intended for educational and informational purposes only. It is not a substitute for professional medical advice, diagnosis, or treatment. Always seek the advice of your physician or other qualified health provider with any questions you may have regarding a medical condition. The author and publisher of this cookbook are not liable for any adverse effects or consequences resulting from the use of the information or recipes contained herein.

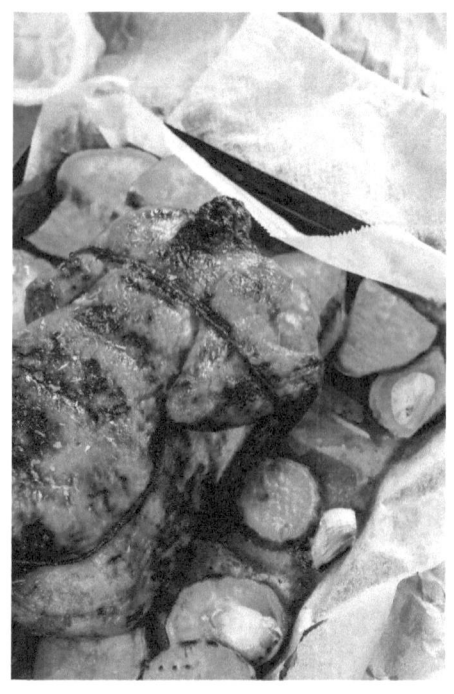

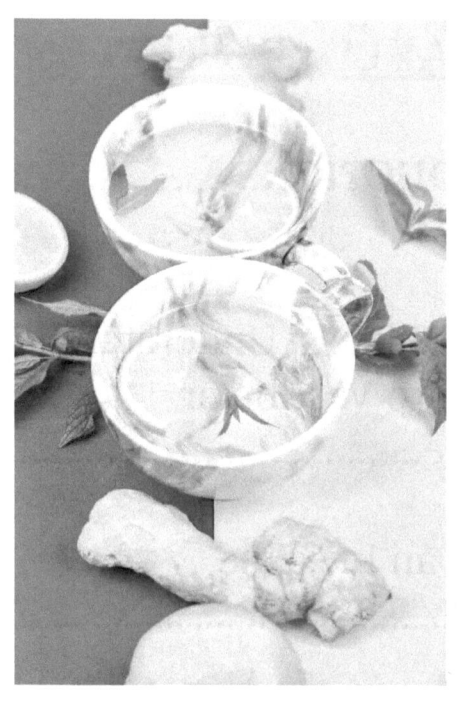

TABLE OF CONTENT

INTRODUCTION..............................13

Invisible Illness: Understanding and Relating to Vestibular Migraine..16

What is an Invisible Illness?..15

Vestibular Migraine: A Primer..17

Understanding the Invisible Nature of Vestibular Migraine...17

Coping Strategies for Invisible Illnesses like Vestibular Migraine...............19

Chapter 1: Understanding Vestibular Migraine..............................21
1.1 What is Vestibular Migraine?...............................22
1.2 Symptoms and Triggers..............................22
1.3 Overview of Migraine Types.................................23
1.4 Causes and Triggers..............................27
1.5 Treatment and Management................................28
1.6 Role of Diet in Management................................33

Chapter 2: Impact of Diet on Vestibular Migraine Episodes..................36
2.1 Effects of Specific Foods and Ingredients......................................36
2.2 Dietary Patterns and Habits..37

2.3 Foods to Include for Symptom Relief.......................................38

Chapter 3: Diagnosing Vestibular Migraine..40
3.1 Understanding the Attack..41
3.2 Symptoms During a Vestibular Migraine Attack..............................42
3.3 Pathophysiology........................43
3.4 Treatment and Management....................................44

Chapters 4: Principles of the Vestibular Migraine Diet..................46
4.1 Identifying Trigger Foods..................46
4.2 Nutritional Guidelines..................48

4.3 Meal Planning Strategies..................49

Chapters 5: Delicious Breakfast Recipes..................52
5.1 Energizing Breakfast Bowls..................52
5.2 Nutrient-Rich Smoothies..................83
5.3 Quick and Easy Morning Fixes..................92

Chapter 6: Lunchtime Favorites..................................96
6.1 Balanced Salads and Dressings.................................97
6.2 Nourishing Soups and Stews.....................................107
6.3 Light and Satisfying Sandwiches..................................126
6.4 Quick Recovery smoothie.....................................154

Chapter 7: Dinner Delights.............................170
7.1 Flavorful and Nourishing Main Courses..............................171
7.2 Comforting Side Dishes..............................180
7.3 One-Pot Meals for Easy Cooking..........................189

Chapter 8: Snacks and Treats..................................202
8.1 Healthy Snack Options...202
8.2 Indulgent Treats with a Purpose..213
8.3 Homemade Energy Bars and Bites...229

Chapter 9: Beverages for Balance..246
9.1 Hydrating Infusions and Teas...246
9.2 Nutrient-Packed Smoothies and Juices..251
9.3 Relaxing Drinks for Evening..252

Chapter 10: Meal Planning and Preparation Tips....................................271

10.1 Creating Weekly Meal Plans..................................271
10.2 Tips for Grocery Shopping......................................273
10.3 Batch Cooking and Freezing Meals..274

Chapter 11: Lifestyle Strategies for Managing Vestibular Migraines......................................276
11.1 Stress Management Techniques..................................278
11.2 Importance of Regular Exercise...279
11.3 Sleep Hygiene Practices..280

Extra bonus : 30-Day Meal Prep Plan..283

Embracing a Balanced Lifestyle with Vestibular Migraines..297
Conclusion......................................301

INTRODUCTION

Welcome to the "*Vestibular Migraine Diet Cookbook*," authored by Anita F. McCluskey This comprehensive guide is dedicated to supporting individuals managing vestibular migraines through dietary choices. Featuring practical solutions and flavorful recipes, this cookbook aims to enhance your health and well-being.

Living with vestibular migraines poses unique challenges that can impact daily life. Anita F. McClukey, drawing from her expertise in nutrition, has curated a selection of recipes designed to alleviate symptoms and promote balance. Each recipe focuses on ingredients known for their potential benefits in managing migraines, ensuring meals are both delicious and supportive.

Whether you're new to managing vestibular migraines or refining your dietary approach, this cookbook offers diverse dishes suitable for various tastes and dietary preferences. From nourishing breakfast ideas to comforting dinners and indulgent treats, every recipe is crafted to prioritize your health and enjoyment.

Within these pages, you'll find practical advice on ingredient choices, meal planning, and adapting recipes to meet individual needs. Anita F. McCluskey's holistic approach emphasizes the role of a balanced diet in migraine management, making this cookbook an essential tool for those embracing mindful eating to take control of their health.

Join us on the path to wellness with the "Vestibular Migraine Diet Cookbook" and discover how simple, nutritious meals can positively impact your life, you are one step to achieving a happy and fulfilling life as you read this book to the very end, not just that but also implementing the step by step in this book in achieving your desired results, now let go.

Invisible Illness: Understanding and Relating to Vestibular Migraine

What is an Invisible Illness?

An invisible illness refers to a medical condition that doesn't exhibit visible signs or symptoms, making it difficult for others to recognize or understand the severity of the condition. These illnesses often impact a person's quality of life, daily functioning, and overall well-being, despite appearing normal on the outside. Examples include chronic pain disorders, autoimmune diseases, mental health conditions, and neurological disorders like vestibular migraine.

Vestibular Migraine: A Primer

Vestibular migraine is a type of migraine headache that includes vestibular symptoms, such as
vertigo, dizziness, balance issues, and visual disturbances. It is characterized by episodes of moderate to severe headaches combined with vestibular symptoms, which can last from a few minutes to several days. Unlike traditional migraines, vestibular migraines are less understood and often misdiagnosed due to their complex symptoms.

Understanding the Invisible Nature of Vestibular Migraine

1. Symptoms : While the headaches in vestibular migraine can be debilitating, the accompanying vestibular symptoms are often less visible but equally disruptive. These include vertigo (a sensation of spinning or movement), sensitivity to light and sound, nausea, and difficulty concentrating.

2. _Impact_ : Individuals with vestibular migraine may experience unpredictable attacks that interfere with daily activities such as work, driving, and social interactions. The unpredictable nature of these symptoms adds to the challenges of managing the condition.

3. _Diagnosis Challenges_ : Due to its overlapping symptoms with other conditions and the absence of visible signs, vestibular migraine can be challenging to diagnose accurately. It often requires a thorough medical history, symptom tracking, and sometimes specialized testing to differentiate it from other vestibular disorders.

Coping Strategies for Invisible Illnesses like Vestibular Migraine

1. *Education and Awareness:* Educating oneself and others about vestibular migraine and invisible illnesses can help reduce misconceptions and promote understanding and support.

2. *Symptom Management:* Developing personalized strategies to manage symptoms, such as stress reduction techniques, dietary changes, and medication, can improve quality of life and reduce the impact of symptoms during flare-ups.

3. *Support Networks:* Connecting with support groups or individuals who understand the challenges of invisible illnesses can provide emotional support and practical tips for coping with daily life.

4. *Advocacy*: Advocating for oneself in healthcare settings and raising awareness in the community can help improve access to appropriate medical care and support services.

Conclusion

Invisible illnesses like vestibular migraine present unique challenges due to their hidden nature and complex symptoms. By raising awareness, promoting understanding, and implementing effective coping strategies, individuals can better manage their condition and improve their overall well-being. Research and ongoing medical advancements are crucial in enhancing diagnosis and treatment options for vestibular migraine and similar conditions, offering hope for better management and quality of life in the future.

Chapters 1: Understanding Vestibular Migraine

In the first chapter, readers are introduced to vestibular migraine, a condition marked by intense episodes of dizziness, vertigo, and heightened sensory sensitivity. The chapter explores how the vestibular system and migraine pathways interact intricately, revealing the neurological foundations of this frequently misunderstood disorder. Through in-depth explanations and real-life case examples, readers gain understanding of the various ways vestibular migraine can manifest and its profound effects on everyday life. From the difficulties in diagnosis to new approaches in treatment, this chapter prepares readers for a thorough exploration of understanding and coping with vestibular migraine.

What is Vestibular Migraine?

Vestibular migraine is a neurological condition marked by recurrent episodes of vertigo, dizziness, and migraines. It is categorized as a type of migraine that predominantly affects the vestibular system, comprising the inner ear and brain regions responsible for processing balance and spatial information.

Symptoms and Triggers

- **Symptoms:** People with vestibular migraine commonly experience:

1. Vertigo: Sensation of spinning or movement while stationary.

2. Dizziness: Feeling lightheaded, unstable, or off-balance.

3. Migraine symptoms: Headaches, sensitivity to light and sound, nausea, and visual disturbances.

4. Motion sensitivity: Heightened sensitivity to motion, particularly during episodes.

Overview of Migraine Types

Migraines are neurological conditions known for severe throbbing head pain, often accompanied by nausea, vomiting, and sensitivity to light and sound. They are classified into different types based on their specific characteristics and triggers. Here's an in-depth exploration:

1. Migraine Without Aura (Common Migraine)

- **Description:** The most common type, marked by intense pain without preceding sensory disturbances.

- **Symptoms:** Throbbing head pain on one side, nausea, vomiting, and sensitivity to light and sound.

- **Duration:** Last from hours to several days.

2. Migraine With Aura (Classic Migraine)

- **Description:** Migraine accompanied or preceded by sensory disturbances known as aura.

- **Aura Symptoms:** Visual disturbances, sensory changes, and speech difficulties.

- **Headache:** Typically follows the aura phase.

3. Chronic Migraine

- **_Description:_** Occurs 15 or more days per month for over three months.

- **_Symptoms:_** Similar to episodic migraines but more frequent and severe.

4. Menstrual Migraine

- **_Description:_** Linked to a woman's menstrual cycle.

- **_Timing:_** Typically occurs around menstruation in most cycles.

5. Vestibular Migraine

- ***Description:*** Involves vertigo or dizziness.

- ***Symptoms:*** Episodes of vertigo, imbalance, and motion sensitivity alongside typical migraine symptoms.

6. Hemiplegic Migraine

- ***Description:*** Rare type with temporary motor weakness on one side of the body.

- ***Symptoms:*** Can resemble stroke-like symptoms.

7. Retinal Migraine

- ***Description:*** Uncommon migraine affecting vision in one eye.

- ***Symptoms:*** Temporary blindness or visual disturbances in one eye.

Causes and Triggers

Migraines can be triggered by various factors including genetics, hormonal changes, stress, certain foods, and sensory stimuli.

Triggers: Various factors can initiate or exacerbate vestibular migraine episodes:

1. Stress: Emotional stress or anxiety.

2. Hormonal changes: Such as those occurring during menstruation or menopause.

3. Environmental factors: Bright lights, loud noises, or strong odors.

4. Physical factors: Fatigue, insufficient sleep, or excessive physical exertion.

5. Certain foods: Such as aged cheeses, processed meats, and foods containing MSG (monosodium glutamate).

Treatment and Management

Effective management often includes medications, lifestyle adjustments, and alternative therapies tailored to individual triggers and symptoms.

Lifestyle Adjustments:

1. Identify Triggers: Record potential triggers such as stress, specific foods, inadequate sleep, or hormonal changes.

2.Dietary Changes: Avoid triggers like caffeine, alcohol, processed foods, and foods containing tyramine (e.g., aged cheese, cured meats).

3.Regular Sleep: Maintain consistent sleep patterns to reduce the frequency of migraine episodes.

4.Stress Reduction: Practice relaxation techniques such as meditation, yoga, or deep breathing exercises.

5. Hydration: Ensure sufficient fluid intake to prevent dehydration, which can provoke migraines.

Medications:

1. Acute Relief: During an attack, medications like triptans (e.g., sumatriptan) or anti-nausea drugs (e.g., metoclopramide) can provide symptom relief.

2. Preventive Medications: For frequent or severe vestibular migraines, doctors may prescribe preventive medications such as beta-blockers (e.g., propranolol), calcium channel blockers (e.g., verapamil), tricyclic antidepressants (e.g., amitriptyline), or anticonvulsants (e.g., topiramate).

Vestibular Rehabilitation Therapy (VRT):

1. Balance Training: VRT focuses on tailored exercises to improve balance and reduce dizziness, overseen by a vestibular therapist.

Alternative Therapies:

1. Acupuncture: Some individuals report relief from acupuncture sessions.

2. Herbal Supplements: Certain herbs like butterbur and feverfew may be helpful, although scientific evidence is limited.

Supportive Measures:

1. Education and Counseling: Understanding vestibular migraines can aid in better management and reduce anxiety associated with attacks.

2. Support Networks: Engaging in support groups or online forums can offer emotional support and practical advice.

Regular Monitoring:

1.Ongoing Evaluation: Regular check-ups with healthcare providers are essential to monitor symptoms, adjust treatments as needed, and ensure overall health.

Emergency Preparedness:

1. Action Plan: Develop a plan with healthcare providers outlining steps to take during severe attacks or sudden worsening of symptoms.

Collaborative Care:

1. Team Approach: Depending on individual needs, collaboration with specialists such as neurologists, otolaryngologists, or physical therapists may be beneficial.

Individuals with vestibular migraines must collaborate closely with healthcare professionals to create a personalized treatment plan addressing their specific triggers and symptoms.

Role of Diet in Management

Diet plays a pivotal role in managing vestibular migraine by identifying and avoiding potential triggers:

- **_Identifying triggers:_** Keeping a food journal to monitor intake and symptoms is crucial.

Common triggers include:

1.Foods rich in tyramine: Such as aged cheeses, cured meats, and fermented foods.

1.MSG (monosodium glutamate): Present in some processed foods, Chinese cuisine, and specific seasonings.

2.Caffeine and alcohol are known to trigger migraines in susceptible individuals.

3.Artificial sweeteners: Studies suggest links between aspartame, sucralose, and migraines.

Recommended dietary practices:

1.Balanced meals: Regular, well-balanced meals aid in stabilizing blood sugar levels and preventing migraines.

2.Adequate hydration: Maintaining proper hydration is essential as dehydration can trigger migraines.

3 Avoidance strategies: Once triggers are identified, consistent avoidance helps reduce the frequency and severity of vestibular migraine episodes.

4.Consultation with healthcare professionals

: Seeking guidance from healthcare providers or registered dietitians ensures personalized dietary recommendations based on individual triggers and overall health.

Conclusion

Managing vestibular migraine involves a comprehensive approach encompassing symptom awareness, trigger identification, and lifestyle adjustments such as dietary modifications. By proactively avoiding triggers and maintaining a healthy lifestyle, individuals can significantly mitigate the impact of vestibular migraine on their daily lives. Regular consultations with healthcare professionals are vital for effective management and improved quality of life.

Chapters 2: Impact of Diet on Vestibular Migraine Episodes

Vestibular migraines lead to recurring bouts of dizziness, vertigo, and occasionally migraines. They are more prevalent among women, and while their precise causes remain unclear, genetics, diet, lifestyle, and surroundings likely play a role. Dietary choices can influence both the frequency and intensity of these episodes.

Effects of Specific Foods and Ingredients

Trigger Foods: Certain foods are known to trigger migraines:

1. Tyramine-rich foods: Examples include aged cheeses, smoked fish, and processed meats.

2. Histamine-rich foods: Such as aged cheeses, alcohol (especially red wine), and fermented foods.

3. Artificial sweeteners: Found in diet sodas and sugar-free products.

4. Caffeine: While it can relieve headaches in moderation, excessive intake or withdrawal can trigger migraines.

2. Food Additives: Additives like MSG, nitrates (found in cured meats), and sulfites (in wine and dried fruits) are reported triggers.

3. Hydration: Inadequate fluid intake can also trigger migraines. Maintaining adequate hydration, primarily through water, is crucial.

Dietary Patterns and Habits

1. Meal Skipping: Irregular meal times or skipping meals can disrupt blood sugar levels, potentially triggering migraines.

2. Low Magnesium Levels: Magnesium deficiency is linked to migraines. Foods rich in magnesium, such as spinach, almonds, and whole grains, may help reduce migraine frequency.

3. High-Sodium Diets: Excessive salt intake can lead to dehydration, which may trigger migraines.

Foods to Include for Symptom Relief

1. Identifying Triggers: Keeping a food diary helps identify specific triggers. Avoiding these triggers can reduce migraine frequency.

2. Balanced Diet: Eating a balanced diet rich in fruits, vegetables, whole grains, lean proteins, and healthy fats supports overall health and may reduce migraines.

3.Hydration: Ensuring sufficient water intake throughout the day helps prevent dehydration-triggered migraines.

4.Regular Eating: Consistent meal times stabilize blood sugar levels, potentially reducing migraine risk.

5.Seeking Professional Advice: Consulting healthcare providers or dietitians specializing in migraine management can provide personalized dietary guidance.

Conclusion

While dietary influences on vestibular migraines vary, understanding and monitoring dietary intake can empower individuals to make informed choices that may help manage and lessen the impact of these episodes.

Chapter 3: Diagnosing Vestibular Migraine

This chapter provides a thorough examination of diagnosing vestibular migraine, a neurological condition characterized by dizziness and vertigo. It discusses the clinical criteria and essential diagnostic methods for differentiating vestibular migraine from other vestibular disorders and migraines with typical aura. Detailed case studies and diagnostic algorithms offer practical insights into the complexities of diagnosis in this area. Furthermore, the chapter underscores the importance of a detailed patient history, symptom assessment, and diagnostic procedures such as vestibular function tests and neuroimaging. By the end of this chapter, readers will gain a comprehensive understanding of the intricate diagnostic approach necessary to accurately identify and differentiate vestibular migraine, crucial for developing effective management and treatment strategies.

Understanding the Attack

Vestibular migraine is a type of migraine characterized by episodes of vertigo, dizziness, and imbalance. Its complex symptoms often mimic other vestibular and neurological disorders, leading to frequent underdiagnosis.

Diagnosis Process

1. *Clinical History*: Patients typically report recurring episodes of vertigo or dizziness lasting from seconds to days, often accompanied by migraine-like headaches.

2. *Diagnostic Criteria*: According to the International Classification of Headache Disorders (ICHD-3), vestibular migraine diagnosis requires:

- Minimum 5 episodes of moderate to severe vertigo lasting 5 minutes to 72 hours.

- Current or past history of migraine with or without aura.

- Vestibular symptoms during at least half of these episodes.

P3.Differential Diagnosis: It's crucial to differentiate vestibular migraine from other causes of vertigo, such as benign paroxysmal positional vertigo (BPPV), Meniere's disease, and other vestibular disorders.

Symptoms During a Vestibular Migraine Attack

During an attack, patients typically experience:

1.Vertigo: A sensation of spinning or movement triggered by head or body position changes.

2. Dizziness: Feeling unsteady or lightheaded.

3. Nausea and Vomiting: Often concurrent with migraine-like headaches.

4. Sensitivity to Light and Sound: Heightened sensitivity to light (photophobia) and sound (phonophobia).

5. Aura: Some may encounter visual disturbances, sensory changes, or language difficulties before or during the attack.

Pathophysiology

The exact mechanisms of vestibular migraine remain incompletely understood but likely involve interactions between the trigeminal and vestibular systems in the brain, alongside cortical spreading depression and neurovascular inflammation.

Treatment and Management

1. Acute Management: Medications such as vestibular suppressants (e.g., meclizine) or antiemetics can alleviate symptoms during attacks.

2. Preventive Therapy: Depending on attack frequency and severity, preventive medications like beta-blockers, calcium channel blockers, and anticonvulsants may be prescribed.

3. Lifestyle Adjustments: Stress reduction, regular sleep, and dietary changes can mitigate triggers and reduce attack frequency.

Prognosis and Outlook

Vestibular migraine is a chronic condition that varies in its impact on quality of life. With proper diagnosis and management, many patients experience significant symptom improvement and reduced attack frequency.

<u>Conclusion</u>

Understanding diagnostic criteria, symptoms, and effective management strategies for vestibular migraine is crucial for healthcare providers. This knowledge aids in accurate diagnosis and enhances treatment outcomes, thereby improving the lives of those affected by this challenging condition.

Chapters 4: Principles of the Vestibular Migraine Diet

Vestibular migraines are a type of migraine that can lead to vertigo, dizziness, and other vestibular symptoms, alongside typical migraine symptoms. Managing these symptoms often requires lifestyle adjustments, including dietary changes. Here are two fundamental principles of the vestibular migraine diet:

4.1 Identifying Trigger Foods

Identifying and avoiding trigger foods is essential for managing vestibular migraines. Trigger foods can vary among individuals, but common culprits include:

1.Foods containing Tyramine: Naturally found in aged cheeses, processed meats, and some fermented foods, tyramine can trigger migraines in susceptible people.

2.Caffeine: While some find relief from migraines with caffeine, others may have migraines triggered by it.

3.Alcohol: Certain types like red wine, beer, and champagne contain compounds that can induce migraines.

4.Artificial additives: MSG (monosodium glutamate) and artificial sweeteners such as aspartame are known triggers for some.

5.Histamine-rich foods: Foods like aged cheeses, smoked meats, and fermented items can contribute to migraines due to histamine intolerance.

Maintaining a detailed food diary can help pinpoint personal triggers. Once identified, these trigger foods should be minimized or avoided to reduce the frequency and severity of vestibular migraine attacks.

4.2 Nutritional Guidelines

A well-balanced diet supports overall health and can potentially lessen the frequency and intensity of vestibular migraines. Key nutritional guidelines include:

1. Hydration: Drinking adequate water throughout the day is crucial to prevent dehydration-triggered migraines.

2. Balanced meals: Regular consumption of balanced meals that incorporate a variety of whole foods—such as fruits, vegetables, whole grains, lean proteins, and healthy fats—helps stabilize blood sugar levels and may prevent migraines.

3. Magnesium-rich foods: Foods like spinach, almonds, and avocados are rich in magnesium, which may help reduce migraines associated with magnesium deficiency.

4. Omega-3 fatty acids: Fatty fish (like salmon and mackerel), flaxseeds, and walnuts contain omega-3s, which have anti-inflammatory properties that could potentially lower migraine frequency.

5. Limiting processed foods: Processed foods often contain additives and preservatives that can trigger migraines in some individuals. Opting for fresh, whole foods whenever possible is advisable.

4.3 Meal Planning Strategies

Effective meal planning can assist individuals with vestibular migraines in maintaining a consistent eating schedule and avoiding trigger foods. Consider these strategies:

1.Planning: Plan meals and snacks ahead of time to ensure balanced nutrition and avoid impulse eating of trigger foods.

2.Batch cooking: Prepare larger quantities of migraine-friendly meals and freeze portions for quick and easy access during migraine episodes.

3.Variety: Rotate through a diverse range of foods to ensure comprehensive nutrient intake and prevent dietary monotony.

4.Consultation with a dietitian: Seeking guidance from a registered dietitian can provide personalized meal plans tailored to individual triggers and nutritional needs.

By adhering to these principles of the vestibular migraine diet—identifying trigger foods, following nutritional guidelines, and employing effective meal planning strategies—individuals can better manage their condition and potentially alleviate the impact of vestibular migraines on daily life. Always consult with healthcare professionals or dietitians before making significant dietary changes, particularly if other health conditions are present.

Chapters 5: Delicious Breakfast Recipes

Welcome to Chapter 5, where we explore a delightful array of breakfast recipes guaranteed to start your day on a delicious note. Whether you're a fan of hearty classics or crave something new and exciting, this chapter has something to satisfy every palate. From fluffy pancakes dripping with syrup to savory omelets bursting with fresh ingredients, each recipe is crafted to bring joy to your morning routine. Dive into these pages and discover the perfect breakfast dish to fuel your day and put a smile on your face.

5.1 Energizing Breakfast Bowls

1. Cinnamon Oat-Meal Muffins

Cinnamon oatmeal muffins sound delicious! They're typically a wholesome treat made with oats, cinnamon, and often include ingredients like applesauce, yogurt, or honey for sweetness.

Ingredients:
- 1 cup rolled oats
- 1 cup all-purpose flour
- 1/2 cup brown sugar (you can adjust this based on your sweetness preference)
- 1 tsp baking powder
- 1/2 tsp baking soda
- 1/2 tsp salt
- 1 tsp ground cinnamon
- 1/2 cup unsweetened applesauce
- 1/4 cup vegetable oil (or melted butter)
- 1/2 cup milk (or almond milk for a dairy-free option)
- 1 large egg
- 1 tsp vanilla extract

Preparation Time: Approximately 15 minutes preparation + 20 minutes baking time.

Nutritional Value: Each muffin (assuming 12 muffins from this recipe) typically contains around 180-200 calories, depending on exact ingredients used. They are generally moderate in calories, with a good balance of carbohydrates, fats, and proteins from oats and milk.

Tips Related to Vestibular Migraine:

1.Avoid Triggers: Some common triggers for vestibular migraines include certain foods (like aged cheeses, processed meats), caffeine, and strong odors. Modify the recipe accordingly to avoid these triggers.

2.Stay Hydrated: Dehydration can trigger migraines, so ensure you drink plenty of water throughout the day.

3.Moderate Caffeine: If caffeine triggers migraines for you, consider using a decaffeinated version of ingredients or reduce the amount of caffeine in your diet.

4.Maintain Regular Meals: Skipping meals or going too long without eating can trigger migraines, so regular and balanced meals, including these muffins, can help stabilize your blood sugar levels.

These muffins can be a delicious and relatively migraine-friendly snack or breakfast option if prepared with attention to your personal triggers. Adjusting ingredients and ensuring hydration and regular eating patterns are key factors in managing vestibular migraines.

2.Vegan Buckwheat pancakes:

"Vegan Bucks" are a vegan adaptation of classic buckwheat pancakes. These pancakes are crafted using buckwheat flour, known for its gluten-free nature and unique nutty taste. Instead of traditional ingredients such as eggs and dairy milk, vegan versions use plant-based substitutes.

To make Vegan Buckwheat pancakes:

Ingredients

1. Buckwheat flour: Provides the base and gives the pancakes their characteristic flavor.

2. Plant-based milk (such as almond milk, soy milk, oat milk): Used instead of dairy milk.

3. Baking powder: To help the pancakes rise.

4. Salt: Enhances flavor.

5. Optional sweetener (like maple syrup or sugar): Adds sweetness if desired.

6.Oil or vegan butter: For cooking the pancakes on a griddle or skillet.

Instructions:

1.In a mixing bowl, combine the buckwheat flour, baking powder, and salt.

2. Add plant-based milk gradually to the dry ingredients, whisking until you achieve a smooth batter consistency.

3.If using a sweetener, add it to the batter and mix well.

4. Heat a non-stick skillet or griddle over medium heat and lightly grease it with oil or vegan butter.

5. Pour a ladleful of batter onto the skillet to form pancakes of your desired size.

6. Cook until bubbles appear on the surface of the pancake and the edges look set (about 2-3 minutes).

7. Flip the pancakes and cook for another 1-2 minutes until golden brown and cooked through.

8. Remove from the skillet and serve warm.

3. Serving:
- Serve Vegan Buckwheat pancakes warm with toppings of your choice such as fresh fruits, maple syrup, vegan whipped cream, or nut butter.

These pancakes are not only delicious but also suitable for those following a vegan diet or looking for a gluten-free option. They provide a wholesome breakfast or brunch option that's satisfying and nutritious.

3. Rotisserie chicken

Rotisserie chicken involves skewering a whole chicken on a spit and roasting it slowly overheating, commonly in an oven or over an open flame. This cooking technique produces moist, tender meat with a crisp outer skin. Typically, the chicken is seasoned or marinated beforehand to enrich its taste. Rotisserie chickens are favored for their convenience and widespread appeal as a ready-to-eat meal option, offering a quick and effortless dining choice. They can be savored alone or incorporated into a variety of dishes such as salads, sandwiches, and soups.

Ingredients:

1. Whole chicken (typically around 3-4 pounds)

2. Seasonings (salt, pepper, herbs like thyme, rosemary, etc.)
3. Optional: Olive oil or butter for basting

Preparation Time:

- ***Preparation time:*** 10-15 minutes (including seasoning)

- ***Cooking time:*** Approximately 1.5 to 2 hours (depending on size and cooking method)

Nutritional Value:
- A typical serving of rotisserie chicken (about 3 ounces, or 85 grams) contains roughly:
- Calories: 170-190
- Protein: 25-30 grams
- Fat: 7-10 grams

- Carbohydrates: 0 grams
- Vitamins and minerals vary, but it's a good source of protein and B vitamins.

Tips:

1. Seasoning: Liberally season the chicken with salt, pepper, and your choice of herbs. You can also add garlic powder, paprika, or lemon zest for extra flavor.

2. Trussing: Trussing (tying up) the chicken helps it cook evenly and keeps the meat moist.

3. Cooking Method: You can roast the chicken in the oven or use a rotisserie attachment on your grill or a specialized rotisserie oven.

4. Basting: Baste the chicken occasionally with its own juices or a mix of olive oil and herbs to keep it moist and flavorful.

5. Internal Temperature: Ensure the chicken reaches an internal temperature of 165°F (74°C) in the thickest part of the meat to ensure it's safely cooked.

6. Resting: Let the chicken rest for 10-15 minutes after cooking to allow the juices to redistribute before carving.

Rotisserie chicken is highly adaptable, perfect on its own with accompanying dishes, shredded for sandwiches, salads, or incorporated into different dishes such as soups and casseroles. Happy cooking!

4. Baked Donut Holes

Baked donut holes are small, round treats that are similar in taste and texture to traditional donuts but are baked instead of fried. They are typically made from a batter similar to that of regular donuts (flour, sugar, eggs, etc.), which is rolled into small balls and baked in a mini muffin tin or on a baking sheet. After baking, they can be coated in sugar, cinnamon, glaze, or other toppings to add flavor and sweetness. Baking instead of frying makes them a bit healthier while still providing that classic donut taste and texture.

Ingredient:

- 1 cup all-purpose flour
- 1/2 cup granulated sugar
- 1 teaspoon baking powder
- 1/4 teaspoon baking soda
- 1/4 teaspoon salt
- 1/2 teaspoon ground cinnamon

- 1/4 cup unsalted butter, melted
- 1/2 cup buttermilk
- 1 teaspoon vanilla extract
- 1 large egg

Preparation Time:
- Preparation: 15 minutes
- Baking: 10-12 minutes
- Total Time: About 30 minutes

Nutritional Value (per serving, makes about 24 donut holes):
- Calories: 70 kcal
- Carbohydrates: 11g
- Fat: 2g
- Protein: 1g
- Sugar: 6g
- Fiber: 0.2g
- Sodium: 70mg

Instructions:

1. Preheat your oven to 350°F (175°C). Grease a mini muffin tin with cooking spray or butter.

2. In a large bowl, whisk together the flour, sugar, baking powder, baking soda, salt, and ground cinnamon.

3. In another bowl, mix together the melted butter, buttermilk, vanilla extract, and egg until well combined.

4. Pour the wet ingredients into the dry ingredients and stir until just combined. Do not overmix; a few lumps are okay.

5. Spoon the batter into the prepared mini muffin tin, filling each cavity about two-thirds full.

6. Bake in the preheated oven for 10-12 minutes, or until the donut holes are lightly golden and a

toothpick inserted into the center comes out clean.

7. Allow the donut holes to cool in the muffin tin for a few minutes, then transfer them to a wire rack to cool completely.

8. Optional: While still warm, you can roll the donut holes in cinnamon sugar (mix 1/2 cup granulated sugar with 1 teaspoon ground cinnamon) for extra flavor.

Enjoy your homemade baked donut holes as a delicious treat!

5. Gluten Free Peach Muffins

Gluten-free peach muffins are muffins that do not contain gluten, such as wheat flour. Instead, they are usually made with alternative flours such as almond flour, rice flour, or a gluten-free flour blend. These muffins are flavored with peach, often using fresh or canned peaches, and may also contain ingredients like eggs, sugar, baking powder, and oil or butter. They are a tasty choice for individuals with gluten sensitivities or celiac disease who wish to indulge in baked treats.

Gluten-free peach muffins, in themselves, are not a specific treatment for vestibular migraines. However, individuals with vestibular migraines or any type of migraine may find that certain dietary adjustments, including avoiding triggers like gluten, can potentially help in managing their symptoms.

1.**_Gluten Sensitivity or Celiac Disease:_** Some people with migraines also have gluten sensitivity or celiac disease. In such cases, consuming gluten can trigger symptoms that may exacerbate migraine attacks. By choosing gluten-free options like gluten-free peach muffins, individuals can potentially reduce the risk of triggering migraines.

2.Dietary Triggers: Migraine triggers vary among individuals, and diet is a common trigger for many. While gluten sensitivity is not universally linked to migraines, some people report improvement in their symptoms when they eliminate gluten from their diet. Therefore, opting for gluten-free foods, such as these muffins, may be part of a broader strategy to manage migraine triggers.

3.Nutritional Content: Peaches themselves contain vitamins and minerals like vitamin C, potassium, and fiber, which are beneficial for overall health. Ensuring a balanced diet that includes nutritious foods can support general well-being, which may indirectly help in managing migraine symptoms.

4.Individual Response: It's important to note that the impact of dietary changes, including going gluten-free, can vary widely among individuals. What works for one person may not work for another. Therefore, if someone suspects that gluten might be a trigger for their migraines, they should consult with a healthcare professional or a registered dietitian for personalized advice.

In summary, while gluten-free peach muffins are not a specific treatment for vestibular migraines, they can be part of a dietary strategy that some individuals find helpful in managing their migraines, particularly if gluten sensitivity or celiac disease is a concern. Consulting with a healthcare provider to determine individual triggers and appropriate dietary adjustments is recommended for those with vestibular migraines or any type of migraine disorder.

Ingredients:

- 1 cup gluten-free flour blend (with xanthan gum)

- 1/2 cup almond flour
- 1/2 cup granulated sugar
- 2 tsp baking powder
- 1/2 tsp baking soda
- 1/4 tsp salt
- 1/2 cup unsweetened applesauce
- 1/4 cup vegetable oil (or melted coconut oil)
- 2 large eggs
- 1 tsp vanilla extract
- 1 cup diced fresh or drained canned peaches

Preparation Time: About 15 minutes

- Nutritional Information: (Per serving - makes 12 muffins)
- Calories: 180 kcal
- Protein: 3g
- Fat: 8g
- Carbohydrates: 24g
- Fiber: 2g

- Sugars: 12g

Instructions:
- Preheat the oven to 375°F (190°C). Grease or line a muffin tin with paper liners.

2. Dry Ingredients:
- Combine gluten-free flour blend, almond flour, sugar, baking powder, baking soda, and salt in a large bowl. Mix well.

3. Wet Ingredients:
- In another bowl, whisk together applesauce, vegetable oil, eggs, and vanilla extract until smooth.

4. Combining:

- Pour wet ingredients into dry ingredients. Stir gently until just combined, avoiding overmixing.

5. Adding Peaches:

- Fold diced peaches into the batter until evenly distributed.

6. Baking:

- Divide batter evenly among muffin cups, filling each about 3/4 full.

7. Bake:
- Bake for 18-20 minutes, or until a toothpick inserted into the center comes out clean.

8. Cooling:

- Let muffins cool in the tin for 5 minutes, then transfer to a wire rack to cool completely.

9. Serve and Store:

- Enjoy warm or at room temperature. Store leftovers in an airtight container at room temperature for up to 3 days, or freeze for longer storage.

These gluten-free peach muffins are moist, flavorful, and make for a delightful breakfast or snack!

6. Quiche Florentine

Quiche Florentine is a classic French dish featuring a rich egg custard blended with spinach (and sometimes other greens like kale) and cheese, all baked in a flaky pie crust. Here's a straightforward recipe to prepare Easy Quiche Florentine:

Ingredients:

- 1 refrigerated pie crust (or homemade, if preferred)
- 5 large eggs
- 1 cup half-and-half (or milk for a lighter version)
- 1 cup shredded cheese (Gruyere, Swiss, or cheddar are good choices)
- 1 package (about 10 oz) frozen chopped spinach, thawed and drained (or fresh spinach, blanched and chopped)
- 1 small onion, finely chopped
- 1 clove garlic, minced (optional)
- Salt and pepper to taste
- Pinch of nutmeg (optional)

Instructions:

1. Preheat Oven and Prepare Crust:
- Heat your oven to 375°F (190°C).
- Fit the pie crust into a 9-inch pie dish, pressing it firmly against the bottom and sides. Trim any excess dough and create a decorative edge.

2. Prepare Filling:

- In a skillet over medium heat, sauté the chopped onion and garlic until softened and translucent (about 5 minutes). Set aside to cool slightly.

- In a large bowl, whisk together eggs, half-and-half (or milk), salt, pepper, and nutmeg until smooth.

- Stir in shredded cheese, drained spinach, and sautéed onion and garlic.

3. Assemble and Bake:

- Pour the egg mixture into the prepared pie crust.

- Place the quiche on a baking sheet to catch any spills and bake for 35-40 minutes, until the center is set and the top is golden brown.

- Allow the quiche to cool for a few minutes before slicing and serving.

Tips:

1.Variations: Enhance with cooked bacon, or ham, or swap cheeses like feta or goat cheese for different flavors.

2.Make Ahead: Prepare ahead and reheat in the oven for convenience.

3.Serving: Ideally warm or at room temperature for brunches, lunches, or dinners paired with a side salad.

Enjoy your Easy Quiche Florentine!

7. Air Fryer Hash Browns

Air fryer hash browns offer a convenient and healthier twist on traditional fried hash browns. Here's a detailed guide to making them:

Understanding Hash Browns:

Hash browns are shredded or grated potatoes usually pan-fried until crispy outside and soft inside, commonly enjoyed as a breakfast side.

Using an Air Fryer:
An air fryer is a kitchen appliance that cooks by circulating hot air around food, mimicking deep frying with less oil for healthier cooking.

Steps to Prepare Air Fryer Hash Browns:

1.Preparation: Begin with frozen hash browns or freshly grated potatoes. Frozen ones are convenient and often pre-seasoned. If using fresh potatoes, grate them using a box grater or food processor, rinsing to remove excess starch.

2. Seasoning: Optionally, season hash browns with salt, pepper, and spices like paprika, garlic powder, or onion powder. Adding chopped onions or bell peppers can enhance flavor.

3. Preheating: Preheat the air fryer to 360-370°F (180-190°C) to ensure even cooking and crispiness.

4. Cooking: Spread hash browns in a single layer in the air fryer basket, adjusting batch size to prevent overcrowding.

5. Air Frying Process: Cook for 10-15 minutes, shaking the basket or flipping halfway through to ensure even crisping.

6. Doneness Check: Hash browns should be golden and crispy. Adjust cooking time based on hash brown thickness and air fryer model.

7. Serving: Once crispy, season to taste and serve immediately as a delightful side dish or breakfast item.

Benefits of Air Fryer Hash Browns:

1. Healthier Choice: Uses less oil than traditional frying, reducing overall fat intake.

2. Crispy Texture: Hot air circulation achieves a crispy exterior while retaining a tender inside.

3. Convenience: Quick and clean preparation compared to frying in a pan.

By following these steps, you can enjoy deliciously crispy hash browns with less oil using your air fryer. Adjust seasoning and cooking times based on personal preference and air fryer specifications for optimal results.

8. Black-Berry Oatmeal Muffins

Black-Berry Oatmeal Muffins are a delightful baked treat that combines the wholesome essence of oats with the sweet-tart flavor of blackberries. Here's how they are typically made:

1. Ingredients: These muffins usually include rolled oats, flour (either whole wheat or all-purpose), a mixture of white and brown sugar, baking powder, baking soda, salt, milk (or buttermilk/yogurt), eggs, melted butter (or oil), vanilla extract, and fresh or frozen blackberries.

Preparation:

1. Dry Ingredients: Mix oats, flour, sugar, baking powder, baking soda, and salt in a bowl.

2.Wet Ingredients: In another bowl, whisk milk, eggs, melted butter, and vanilla extract.

3.Combining: Gently fold the wet ingredients into the dry mixture until just blended. Avoid overmixing; a few lumps are okay.

3.Adding Blackberries: Carefully fold in fresh or thawed frozen blackberries. Coating them lightly in flour beforehand can help prevent them from sinking in the muffin batter.

3. Baking:

- Spoon the batter into muffin cups lined with paper liners or grease.

- Bake in a preheated oven at 375°F (190°C) for about 18-20 minutes, or until a toothpick inserted into the center comes out clean.

4. Cooling and Serving:

- Let the muffins cool in the pan for a few minutes before transferring them to a wire rack to cool completely.

- Enjoy warm or at room temperature.

These muffins are widely enjoyed for breakfast or as a snack, offering a blend of fiber from oats and the antioxidant-rich flavor of blackberries. They are typically moist and slightly dense due to the oats, with bursts of fruity goodness from the blackberries.

5.2 Nutrient-Rich Smoothies

9. Apple Carrots smoothie

An Apple Carrot smoothie usually mixes fresh apples and carrots with ingredients such as orange juice, ginger, or yogurt to enhance its taste and consistency. It's renowned for its health benefits, offering ample vitamins A and

C from the carrots and apples. Variants may incorporate honey for sweetness or cinnamon for added flavor. This smoothie provides a delicious and easy way to enjoy a fusion of fruits and vegetables.

A smoothie containing apple and carrots can be beneficial for individuals dealing with vestibular migraines for several reasons:

1.Rich in Essential Nutrients: Apples and carrots are packed with vitamins such as C and A, minerals like potassium, and antioxidants. These nutrients support overall health and may help in reducing the frequency and intensity of migraines.

2.Promotes Hydration: Both ingredients have high water content, aiding in hydration. Dehydration is a common migraine trigger, so maintaining adequate hydration levels can help prevent attacks.

3.Anti-inflammatory Properties: Apples and carrots contain compounds known for their anti-inflammatory properties. Since chronic inflammation is often linked to migraines, consuming these foods may assist in managing symptoms.

4.Stabilizes Blood Sugar Levels: The natural sugars in apples and carrots provide sustained energy release without causing spikes in blood sugar levels. This stability can help in avoiding fluctuations that might trigger migraines.

5.Supports Digestive Health: High in dietary fiber, apples and carrots promote healthy digestion. Many migraine sufferers experience exacerbated symptoms from digestive issues, making a smoothie that aids gut health beneficial.

6.Ease of Digestion: Smoothies are generally easier on the digestive system compared to solid foods, which is advantageous during migraine attacks when nausea and sensitivity are common.

While incorporating nutritious foods like apples and carrots into your diet can potentially reduce migraine frequency and severity, individual responses may vary. It's important to monitor how these foods affect your specific migraine triggers and symptoms. For personalized advice and treatment recommendations, consulting with a healthcare professional is recommended.

Ingredients:

- 1 apple, cored and chopped
- 1 large carrot, peeled and chopped
- 1 cup of unsweetened almond milk (or any milk of your choice)

- 1 tablespoon of honey or maple syrup (optional, for sweetness)
- 1/2 teaspoon of ground cinnamon (optional, for flavor)

Preparation Time:
- Approximately 5 minutes

Nutritional Value:
- Calories: Around 150 kcal
- Carbohydrates: 35g
- Fiber: About 7g
- Protein: Around 2g
- Fat: Less than 1g
- Vitamin A: Provides over 200% of daily recommended intake
- Vitamin C: Provides about 15% of daily recommended intake

Instructions:

1. Prepare the ingredients: Wash the apple and carrot thoroughly. Core the apple and peel the carrot, then chop them into smaller pieces.

2. Blend: In a blender, combine the chopped apple, carrot, almond milk, honey or maple syrup (if using), and ground cinnamon (if using).

3. Blend until smooth: Blend on high speed until the mixture is smooth and well combined. If the consistency is too thick, you can add a bit more almond milk or water to achieve your desired thickness.

4. Serve: Pour the smoothie into glasses and optionally garnish with a sprinkle of cinnamon on top. Serve immediately and enjoy!

This smoothie is not only delicious but also packed with nutrients from the apple and carrot, providing a good mix of vitamins and fiber to start your day or to enjoy as a refreshing snack.

10. Bananas Applesauce Muffins

Banana Applesauce Muffins are a type of muffin made primarily with ripe bananas and unsweetened applesauce.

1. Ingredients:

- 1 and 1/2 cups all-purpose flour
- 1 teaspoon baking powder
- 1 teaspoon baking soda
- 1/2 teaspoon salt
- 1 teaspoon ground cinnamon
- 1/2 cup unsweetened applesauce

- 1/2 cup mashed ripe bananas (about 2 medium bananas)
- 1/2 cup brown sugar (you can adjust to taste)
- 1/4 cup melted butter or vegetable oil
- 1/4 cup milk (dairy or non-dairy)
- 1 teaspoon vanilla extract
- Optional: 1/2 cup chopped nuts (like walnuts or pecans), chocolate chips, or dried fruit

These ingredients will give you moist and flavorful Banana Applesauce Muffins. Enjoy baking!

Preparation:

1.Prepare Wet Ingredients: Mash the bananas until smooth. In a separate bowl, combine mashed bananas with applesauce, eggs, vanilla extract, and sweetener.

2. Prepare Dry Ingredients: In another bowl, mix flour, baking powder, baking soda, and salt.

3. Combine: Gradually blend the dry ingredients into the wet mixture until just combined. Avoid over mixing to keep the muffins light.

3. Baking:

1. Preheat Oven: Typically to 350°F (175°C).

- **Fill Muffin Cups:** Spoon batter into lined or greased muffin cups, filling each about 3/4 full.
- **2. Bake:** Bake for 18-20 minutes until a toothpick inserted into the center comes out clean or with a few crumbs.

4. Variations: Customize with additions like nuts, chocolate chips, or spices such as cinnamon or nutmeg for added flavor.

5. Health Benefits: These muffins are often considered healthier due to less added sugar and fat, relying on the natural sweetness of bananas and applesauce.

In summary, Banana Applesauce Muffins are moist, flavorful, and a great way to enjoy a baked treat while incorporating fruit.

11. Quick and Easy Morning Fixes

Starting your day with suitable foods can positively impact vestibular migraine symptoms. Here are some nutritious, migraine-friendly morning options that are quick and simple to prepare:

1. Nutrient-Packed Smoothie:

Blend spinach, banana, Greek yogurt, and berries for a refreshing smoothie. Spinach provides magnesium, bananas offer potassium, and berries are rich in antioxidants.

2. Overnight Oats:

Combine oats, chia seeds, almond milk, and honey in a jar and refrigerate overnight. Top with fresh fruits and nuts in the morning. Oats are high in fiber and help stabilize blood sugar levels.

3. Avocado Toast Variation:

Spread mashed avocado on whole-grain toast and top with tomatoes and pumpkin seeds. Avocados provide healthy fats and potassium, while whole grains offer sustained energy.

4. Protein-Packed Egg Bowl:

Scramble eggs with spinach and mushrooms, and serve with whole-grain toast. Eggs are rich in protein and B vitamins, beneficial for neurological health.

5. Yogurt Parfait:

Layer Greek yogurt with granola and fresh fruits for a nutritious parfait. Greek yogurt supplies protein, calcium, and probiotics, supporting gut health and overall well-being.

These morning fixes are quick, delicious, and packed with nutrients that support a diet suitable for managing vestibular migraines. Starting your day with these options can help alleviate symptoms and promote overall health.

Conclusion:

Incorporating these quick and easy morning fixes into your routine can significantly aid in managing vestibular migraine symptoms. Adjust your diet based on individual triggers and preferences, and consider consulting a healthcare professional or registered dietitian specializing in migraine management for personalized guidance. By taking a proactive approach to nutrition and lifestyle, you can effectively manage vestibular migraines and improve your overall well-being.

Chapter 6: Lunchtime Favorites

Chapter 6 of "Lunchtime Favorites" presents a delightful selection of recipes aimed at transforming lunch into a memorable experience. This section emphasizes dishes that are not just tasty but also practical for midday meals at home, work, or on the move. From flavorful sandwiches to refreshing salads bursting with fresh ingredients, each recipe is designed to satisfy cravings and provide nourishment during the busiest part of the day. Whether you're in search of quick and simple options or more elaborate dishes to impress, Chapter 6 of "Lunchtime Favorites" caters to diverse tastes and occasions, ensuring lunchtime is eagerly anticipated and thoroughly enjoyed.

6.1 Balanced Salads and Dressings

Certainly! "Balanced salads and dressings" refer to salads that are nutritionally complete, containing a variety of ingredients such as leafy greens, vegetables, proteins (like grilled chicken or tofu), healthy fats (such as avocado or nuts), and carbohydrates (like whole grains or fruits).

The dressing is essential for harmonizing flavors and textures while supplying healthy fats or oils that aid in absorbing fat-soluble vitamins from the vegetables. It's important to opt for dressings made from nutritious oils such as olive oil and to use them sparingly to manage calorie intake.

In summary, balanced salads and dressings are not only tasty but also provide a broad spectrum of nutrients that support a healthy lifestyle.

1. Balanced Salad:

A balanced salad typically includes a variety of ingredients that offer a blend of nutrients, tastes, textures, and colors. Here's what usually comprises a balanced salad:

1. Leafy Greens: These form the salad's base and provide vitamins, minerals, and fiber. Common choices are spinach, kale, arugula, and mixed lettuces.

2. Protein: Adding protein boosts the salad's filling and nutritional value. Options include grilled chicken, tofu, beans (such as chickpeas or black beans), quinoa, eggs, or seafood like shrimp or salmon.

3. Vegetables: Colorful vegetables contribute crunch, flavor, and essential vitamins and minerals. Common selections are tomatoes, cucumbers, bell peppers, carrots, onions, and radishes.

4. Fruit (optional): Adding fruits like berries, apples, or citrus segments can impart sweetness and additional nutrients such as antioxidants and vitamins.

5. Healthy Fats: Sources such as avocado, nuts (like almonds, walnuts), seeds (such as pumpkin or sunflower seeds), or a drizzle of olive oil provide beneficial fats that support heart health and satiety.

6. Dressing: A light dressing made from olive oil, balsamic vinegar, lemon juice, or yogurt-based dressings ties the salad together, adding flavor without excess calories.

7. Extras (optional): Ingredients like cheese (feta, goat cheese), croutons (preferably whole grain), or dried fruits can enhance texture and flavor, but should be used sparingly to maintain the salad's balance.

Balanced salads are not only delicious but also offer a wide array of nutrients, making them a healthy and satisfying meal choice. Adjusting ingredient quantities according to personal taste and nutritional preferences can further optimize the salad's balance.

Preparation Time: Approximately 15 minutes

Ingredients:
- Mixed greens (such as spinach, arugula, and lettuce)
- Cherry tomatoes
- Sliced cucumber
- Diced bell peppers
- Sliced avocado
- Grilled chicken breast, sliced (optional)

Instructions:

1. Prepare and wash all vegetables.
2. Combine mixed greens, cherry tomatoes, cucumber, bell peppers, and avocado in a large salad bowl.
3. Add grilled chicken slices if desired.

Certainly! Here's an example of the nutritional information for a well-balanced salad:

Nutrition Facts per Serving:
- Calories: 250 kcal
- Total Fat:15 grams
- Saturated Fat: 2 grams
- Trans Fat: 0 grams
- Cholesterol:r 0 milligrams
- Sodium: 300 milligrams
- Total Carbohydrates: 25 grams
- Dietary Fiber: 8 grams

- Sugars: 10 grams
- Protein: 10 grams

2. Lemon Vinaigrette Dressing:

Lemon vinaigrette dressing is a straightforward and adaptable blend primarily comprising lemon juice, olive oil, and seasonings. Here's a fundamental breakdown of its ingredients and preparation:

1. Lemon Juice: This essential element provides a zesty, citrusy flavor. Freshly squeezed lemon juice is typically preferred for its vibrant and clean taste.

2. Olive Oil: Serving as the dressing's foundation, olive oil contributes a smooth texture and a hint of richness. Extra virgin olive oil is commonly chosen for its robust flavor.

3. Seasonings: To enhance the taste, salt and pepper are frequently added. Sometimes, a dash of Dijon mustard is included to both emulsify the dressing and deepen its flavor profile.

4. Optional Herbs and Garlic: Additional ingredients like minced garlic, fresh herbs such as parsley or thyme, or even a touch of honey can be incorporated to add complexity to the flavor.

Preparation:

1. Basic Ratio: A typical guideline is one part lemon juice to three parts olive oil, though this can be adjusted according to personal taste.

2. *Emulsification*: Begin by whisking together the lemon juice and, if desired, mustard. Gradually drizzle in the olive oil while whisking vigorously to achieve a smooth, emulsified consistency.

2. *Seasoning*: Adjust the seasoning with salt, pepper, and any other desired spices to taste. Modify the acidity level by adding more lemon juice if necessary.

3. *Storage*: Store any unused dressing in a sealed container in the refrigerator. Before using, allow it to reach room temperature and shake or whisk it to recombine.

***Usage*:**
1. Lemon vinaigrette is versatile and complements various salads, including mixed greens, pasta salads, or grilled vegetables.

2. It pairs well with seafood, chicken, or can be used as a marinade for meats.

In summary, lemon vinaigrette is appreciated for its refreshing, tangy flavor and its ability to enhance a wide array of dishes with its bright acidity and subtle olive oil base.

Ingredients:
- 1/4 cup olive oil
- 2 tablespoons fresh lemon juice
- 1 teaspoon Dijon mustard
- 1 clove garlic, minced
- Salt and pepper to taste

Instructions:
1. Whisk together olive oil, lemon juice, Dijon mustard, minced garlic, salt, and pepper in a small bowl until well blended.
2. Adjust seasoning as per taste preference.

Serving:

- Just before serving, drizzle the lemon vinaigrette dressing over the salad.

- Gently toss to ensure even coating.

- Enjoy your nutritious and balanced salad!

Nutritional Information (per serving, approximate):

- Calories: 120 kcal
- Total Fat: 13 g (Saturated Fat: 1.5 g, Trans Fat: 0 g)
- Cholesterol: 0 mg
- Sodium: 150 mg
- Total Carbohydrates: 2 g (Dietary Fiber: 0 g, Sugars: 1 g)
- Protein: 0 g

Note: Nutritional values may vary depending on the specific ingredients used.

Preparation Time:
- Preparation: 5 minutes
- Total Time: 5 minutes

This Lemon Vinaigrette recipe typically involves combining lemon juice, olive oil, Dijon mustard, garlic, salt, and pepper and whisking thoroughly. Adjust ingredient amounts to match your taste preferences.

4 Recipes:

6.2 Nourishing Soups and Stews

"Nourishing soups and stews" are hearty and wholesome meals prepared by gently cooking a variety of ingredients such as vegetables, meats, legumes, and spices in a tasty broth or sauce. These dishes are prized for their comforting qualities and nutritional benefits, offering a blend of proteins, vitamins, and minerals. They can be adapted with different ingredients to match individual tastes and dietary needs, making them adaptable choices for meals, especially during colder times of the year.

1. Chicken and Vegetable Soup

- **_Ingredients:_** Chicken breast, carrots, celery, potatoes, low-sodium chicken broth, fresh thyme and parsley, salt, pepper.

- **_Method:_** Cook chicken with vegetables in broth until tender. Season with herbs, salt, and pepper.

2. Ginger Turmeric Carrot Soup

- **_Ingredients:_** Carrots, ginger, turmeric, coconut milk, vegetable broth, onion, garlic, olive oil, salt, pepper.

- **_Method:_** Sauté onion and garlic, add carrots, ginger, turmeric, broth. Simmer until carrots are soft, blend until smooth, stir in coconut milk, season.

3. Salmon and Spinach Chowder

- **_Ingredients:_** Salmon filets, spinach, potatoes, leeks, dill, low-fat milk, chicken broth, olive oil, salt, pepper.

- **_Method:_** Sauté leeks, potatoes in broth and milk until tender. Add salmon, spinach, dill, simmer until salmon flakes. Season to taste.

4. Quinoa and Vegetable Stews

- **_Ingredients:_** Quinoa, mixed vegetables (bell peppers, zucchini, tomatoes),

vegetable broth, onion, garlic, olive oil, cumin, paprika, salt, pepper.
- **_Method:_** Sauté onion, garlic, add vegetables, quinoa, broth, spices. Simmer until quinoa is cooked and vegetables are tender. Adjust seasoning.

5. Miso Soup with Tofu and Seaweed

- **_Ingredients_**: Miso paste, tofu, seaweed (wakame), green onions, low-sodium vegetable broth, soy sauce.

- **_Method:_** Dissolve miso paste in broth, add tofu, seaweed, simmer until heated through. Garnish with green onions.

6. Lentil and Kale Soup

- **_Ingredients:_** Brown lentils, kale, carrots, celery, onion, garlic, vegetable broth, olive oil, bay leaf, thyme, salt, pepper.

- **_Method:_** Sauté onion, garlic, add lentils, broth, vegetables, herbs. Simmer until lentils are tender. Adjust seasoning, stir in kale until wilted.

These soup and stew recipes are crafted to be soothing, gentle on the stomach, and packed with nutrients, making them ideal for managing symptoms during vestibular migraine episodes.

7. Chicken And Brown Rice Soup

This chicken and brown rice soup is perfect for a comforting, effortless, and snug meal ideal for a straightforward yet hearty dinner or lunch. It's naturally free of gluten and dairy, with basic ingredients that evoke the essence of a traditional chicken soup, while fresh herbs enrich it with a more robust and delightful taste.

Ingredients:

- 1 tablespoon olive oil

- 2 garlic cloves, minced

- 2 shallots, finely chopped

- 2 celery ribs, chopped

- 2 large carrots, chopped or about 10 baby carrots chopped

- 1 teaspoon kosher salt

- ⅔ cup brown rice

- 1 bay leaf

- 1 bouquet garni - a few sprigs of fresh thyme and rosemary tied together with kitchen twine

- 5-6 cups vegetable or chicken broth

- 1-2 cups water
- 1 rotisserie chicken meat, lightly chopped

- fresh black pepper to taste

Instructions:

1. Heat olive oil in a large, sturdy pot over medium heat. Add garlic, shallots, celery, carrots, and kosher salt. Cook, stirring occasionally until softened and fragrant, about

5-6 minutes. Be careful not to brown the garlic. Add rice, bay leaf, and bouquet garni, and mix well. Pour in 5 cups of chicken broth and 1 cup of water. Bring to a gentle simmer, cover with a lid.

2. After 35 minutes of covered cooking, check if the rice is fully cooked. Remove the bouquet garni and stir in chopped rotisserie chicken. Adjust consistency by adding another cup of water or broth if desired. I prefer using 5 cups of broth and 2 cups of water for a balanced flavor.

3. Simmer briefly, adjust seasoning with more kosher salt and freshly ground black pepper to taste. Serve warm or refrigerate until ready to serve. Note that the soup will thicken over time, so adjust thickness before serving by adding more water or broth as needed.

Nutrition Facts (per serving):

- Serving size: 12oz
- Energy: 456 calories
- Macronutrients:
- Carbs: 30g
- Protein: 47g
- Fat: 16g
- Vitamins and Minerals:
- Vitamin A: 3880IU
- Vitamin C: 2mg
- Calcium: 46mg
- Iron: 2mg
- Other nutrients:
- Fiber: 2g
- Sugar: 3g
- Sodium: 1746 mg
- Potassium: 640mg
- Cholesterol: 154mg"

8:*Lemongrass Ginger Soup*

This lemongrass ginger soup recipe uses spices that can ease migraines and fight inflammation.

You can easily swap shrimp for rotisserie chicken, and choose pasta or farro instead of butternut squash.

Ingredients:

- 1 2-3 lb spaghetti squash, cut in half with seeds and pulp scooped out

- 1 lb uncooked, peeled and deveined shrimp Get the tail off to make your life easier

- 2 stalks of lemongrass

- 3 garlic cloves, peeled and sliced

- 3 inch ginger piece, peeled and sliced

- 2 tablespoon ghee or olive oil

- ¼ cup cilantro, chopped

- 2 green onions, chopped

- 6 cups vegetable or chicken broth Try my HYH safe instant pot chicken broth!

- kosher salt to taste

Instruction

1. Begin by preheating your oven to 400 degrees Fahrenheit. Apply olive oil to the cut sides of the spaghetti squash halves and season them with salt and pepper. Place them with the cut side down on a baking sheet and bake for approximately 50 minutes. Once baked, remove them and allow them to cool slightly. Use a fork to shred the flesh into strands resembling spaghetti.

2. While the squash is baking, prepare the lemongrass by trimming the ends, halving each stalk, and cutting them into 3-inch segments. In

a large pot, melt butter or heat olive oil. Add garlic, lemongrass, and ginger, and cook over medium heat for about 2 minutes until aromatic.

3. Pour broth into the pot and bring it to a boil. Lower the heat and let it simmer for 30 minutes. Strain the broth through a fine sieve and return it to the pot. Add shrimp or chicken and simmer for an additional 10 minutes.

4. Mix the shredded spaghetti squash with green onions and cilantro in a bowl. Pour the prepared broth over the vegetables and serve promptly.

Preparation time:

- **_SoupCuisine:_** Healthy Prep Time: 15minutes

- ***Cook Time:*** 50minutes

- ***Total Time:*** 1hour

- ***hour 5 Servings:*** 4 people Calories:

Nutritional information
- Energy: 248 calories
- Carbohydrates: 7 grams
- Protein: 31 grams
- Fat: 11 grams
- Saturated Fat: 6 grams
- Cholesterol: 305 milligrams
- Sodium: 990 milligrams
- Potassium: 461 milligrams
- Fiber: 1 gram
- Sugar: 1 gram
- Vitamin A: 127 IU
- Vitamin C: 7 milligrams
- Calcium: 187 milligrams
- Iron: 3 milligrams

9. Boursin Broccoli Soup

Boursin Broccoli Soup is a creamy and flavorful soup made primarily with broccoli and Boursin cheese.

Ingredients:

- 1/4 cup butter
- 2 large shallots, finely chopped
- 2 large carrots, finely chopped (1 cup)
- 1/4 cup all-purpose flour (use gluten-free if necessary)
- 3 cups vegetable broth
- 1 1/2 cups whole milk*
- 1 head of broccoli, cut into florets (about 2 cups florets)
- 5 oz Boursin Garlic & Herb cheese
- 3/4 teaspoon kosher salt (optional for lower sodium)
- 1/2 teaspoon black pepper

Preparation Time: 10 minutes

- Cooking Time: 20 minutes

- Total Time: 30 minutes
- Servings: 4
- Calories per serving: 418

Instructions:

1. Melt butter in a large, sturdy pot over medium heat. Add diced shallots and carrots, cooking for about 2 minutes until they're fragrant and slightly soft, stirring often.

2. Sprinkle ¼ cup of flour over the vegetables, stirring to coat evenly. Gradually add ½ cup of broth, whisking until the mixture is smooth and the flour is fully blended.

3. Pour in the rest of the broth and whole milk. Bring the mixture to a gentle simmer (be cautious not to boil to prevent curdling) and cook for 8-10 minutes until it thickens slightly.

4. Add broccoli florets and cook for an additional 5 minutes until they become tender.

5. Remove the pot from the heat and stir in Boursin cheese until the soup is creamy and smooth. Taste and adjust seasoning with salt and pepper to your liking.

Nutritional information:
- Energy: 418 calories
- Carbohydrates: 29g
- Protein: 12g
- Fat: 30g
- Saturated Fat: 19g
- Trans Fat: 1g
- Cholesterol: 76mg
- Sodium: 434mg
- Potassium: 756 mg
- Fiber: 6g
- Sugars: 12g
- Vitamin A: 6913 IU
- Vitamin C: 138 mg

- Calcium: 220mg
- Iron: 2mg

10. Vegetarian Tortilla Soup

"Vegetarian Tortilla Soup is a nourishing and flavorful dish that combines a variety of vegetables, beans, and tortillas in a savory broth.

Ingredients list:
- Olive oil
- Shallots
- Sweet potatoes
- Frozen corn
- Jalapeno pepper
- Garlic
- Ground cumin

- Chili powder (or Chipotle powder for extra heat)
- Black beans (canned)
- Diced tomatoes (canned)
- Vegetable broth
- Fresh cilantro
- White vinegar
- Salt
- Optional toppings: corn chips or tortillas"

This comforting soup is:
- Filling and satisfying
- Rich in flavor and nutrients
- Diverse in texture, with crunchy vegetables and soft tortillas
- Customizable with your favorite toppings like avocado, sour cream, or cheese
- It's a great meatless option that's both delicious and nutritious!"

Instructions:

1. Heat oil in a large pot over medium heat. Add shallots, sweet potatoes, corn, jalapeno, and salt. Cook, stirring often, until the vegetables soften (5-7 minutes).
2. Add garlic, chili powder, and cumin. Cook, stirring, until fragrant (1 minute).
3. Add black beans, diced tomatoes, and vegetable broth. Stir to combine.
4. Bring the mixture to a low simmer (small bubbles around the edges). Cook, without boiling, until the potatoes soften (25-30 minutes).
5. Season to taste, add vinegar and cilantro.
6. Serve with tortilla chips or make your own by baking tortilla strips in the oven until lightly browned (7-9 minutes).

"Nourishment Facts:

- Energy: 398 calories
- Macronutrients:
- Carbs: 76g

- Protein: 18g
- Fat: 8g
- Vitamins and Minerals:
- Vitamin A: 16417IU
- Vitamin C: 22mg
- Calcium: 157 mg
- Iron: 7mg
- Other nutrients:
- Fiber: 21g
- Sugar: 9g
- Sodium: 331mg
- Potassium: 1385mg

6.3 Light and Satisfying Sandwiches

Light and satisfying sandwiches are typically known for their blend of flavors, textures, and nutritional value. Here's a breakdown of how these sandwiches are usually composed:

1. Bread: Opt for whole grain or whole wheat varieties for their fiber and nutrient content, which are lighter than traditional white bread. Alternatively, wraps or pitas offer diversity.

2. Protein: Select lean proteins like grilled chicken breast, turkey, tuna, or tofu. These choices are lower in fat and calories compared to processed meats such as salami or bacon.

3. Vegetables: Include plenty of fresh vegetables such as lettuce, spinach, cucumber, tomatoes, bell peppers, and sprouts for their crunch, flavor, and nutritional benefits. They add bulk and fiber without excess calories.

4. Condiments: Use light spreads such as hummus, mustard, or Greek yogurt-based dressings instead of heavy mayonnaise or creamy sauces. These options provide flavor with fewer calories and less saturated fat.

5. Cheese (optional): If desired, opt for lighter cheeses like part-skim mozzarella or feta. These add taste without adding unnecessary calories.

6. Extras: Enhance flavor and texture with herbs, spices, or a splash of vinegar or lemon juice. These additions elevate taste without significantly increasing the calorie count.

Creating a sandwich that is both light and satisfying involves selecting ingredients that are nutritious and flavorful without being overly heavy or calorie-dense. This ensures a balanced meal that keeps you feeling full and energized without any heaviness.

1. Goat Cheese Sandwich with Arugula And Cucumber

A Goat Cheese Sandwich with Arugula and Cucumber typically includes the following:

1.Bread: Often a crusty artisan or hearty whole grain bread is used.

2.Goat Cheese: Known for its creamy texture and distinct flavor, it spreads easily for sandwiches.

3. Arugula: This peppery, leafy green adds a fresh, slightly bitter contrast to the creamy goat cheese.

4. Cucumber: Thinly sliced for a crisp, refreshing crunch.

5.Optional Ingredients: Sometimes includes sliced tomatoes, a drizzle of balsamic glaze or honey, or a sprinkle of black pepper for added flavor.

Preparation:

1. Toast Bread: Optionally lightly toast for texture.

2. Spread Goat Cheese: Generously apply to one or both slices of bread.

3. Layer Ingredients: Arrange arugula evenly on one slice, and top with cucumber slices.

4. Assemble: Close the sandwich and press gently to secure it.

5. Serve: Cut as desired and serve immediately.

Tips:

- **Variations:** Customize with ingredients like roasted red peppers or avocado.

- **Texture:** Use thinly sliced cucumber to blend flavors well.

- **_Pairing_**: Ideal with soup or salad for a complete meal.

This combination of creamy goat cheese, peppery arugula, and crisp cucumber creates a refreshing and satisfying sandwich, perfect for a light meal.

Ingredients
- 2 slices of sandwich bread
- 9 thinly sliced seedless English cucumbers
- Small handful of arugula
- 1 ounce of fresh goat cheese
- 2-3 teaspoons of sweet chili jam

Instructions:
1.Spread goat cheese on one slice of bread and apply sweet chili jam or sauce on the other slice.

2.Add cucumber and arugula, then put the sandwich together and enjoy!

Nutritional information:

Each sandwich serving provides 236 calories, consisting of 29 g carbohydrates, 10g protein, and 8g fat (including 4g saturated fat). It also contains 13 mg cholesterol, 449 mg sodium, and 58 mg potassium, with 1g fiber and 8g sugar. Additionally, it supplies 293 IU Vitamin A, 170 mg calcium, and 2 mg iron.

2. Crustless Chicken Pot Pie

A Chicken Pot Pie is a variation of the classic dish that skips the usual flaky pastry topping. Here's how it typically differs and why it's prepared this way:

1. *No Pastry Crust:* Instead of the traditional flour, butter, and water crust, this version focuses solely on the savory filling. This adjustment reduces carbs and makes the dish lighter.

2. Focus on Filling: The filling stars diced or shredded chicken, mixed vegetables like peas, carrots, and sometimes corn, all bathed in a creamy sauce thickened with flour or cornstarch. It's seasoned generously with herbs and spices for maximum flavor.

3. Health Considerations: Crustless pot pies appeal to those cutting carbs or avoiding gluten, as traditional crusts use wheat flour. This version is also lighter in calories and fat without the buttery crust.

4. Cooking Method: The filling ingredients are typically cooked on the stovetop or baked in a casserole until flavors meld and the mixture thickens. Serve it piping hot from the oven or cool it a bit before enjoying it.

5. Variations: Like its classic counterpart, there are endless variations of crustless chicken pot pie. Recipes may vary the vegetables, swap meets, or adjust sauces to suit different tastes and diets.

In essence, a crustless chicken pot pie delivers the comforting flavors of the original without the pastry, making it ideal for those seeking a lighter or gluten-free option.

Ingredients:
- 1 pound boneless chicken breast, diced
- 2 teaspoons olive oil
- Salt and pepper
- ¼ cup butter
- 2 tablespoons all-purpose flour
- 2 shallots, finely chopped
- 2 large carrots, diced (about ¾ cup)
- ½ cup frozen peas
- ½ cup frozen corn
- 1 cup whole milk
- 1 ¼ cups vegetable or chicken broth
- ¼ teaspoon dried thyme
- ½ cup panko breadcrumbs

Instructions:

1. Cut chicken breast into small pieces and season with kosher salt and pepper. Heat olive oil in a large, deep pan over medium heat. Cook chicken for approximately 3 minutes on each side until browned and fully cooked. Remove chicken from the pan and set aside.

2. In the same pan, add 1 tablespoon of butter, chopped shallots, and carrots. Cook over medium-low heat until softened, about 5 minutes. Add peas, corn, and the remaining butter. Stir in 2 tablespoons of flour until vegetables are coated.

3. Pour in broth and simmer gently for 1-2 minutes, stirring to ensure the flour blends smoothly. Gradually add milk as the mixture thickens. Season with thyme, salt, and pepper to taste. Simmer for 8-10 minutes, stirring

frequently, until the sauce coats the back of a spoon. Add the cooked chicken back into the pan.

4. Spoon the chicken pot pie filling into individual oven-safe ramekins. Sprinkle with panko breadcrumbs and broil on high for about 1 minute until lightly browned. Serve hot.

Nutritional information:

- **_Energy:_** 380 calories

- **_Carbs:_** 25 grams

- **_Protein:_** 31 grams

- **_Fat:_** 18 grams (Saturated Fat: 9g)

- **_Cholesterol:_** 109 milligrams

- **_Sodium:_** 361 milligrams

- **_Potassium:_** 822 milligrams

- **_Fiber:_** 3 grams

- **_Sugar:_** 7 grams

- **_Vitamin A:_** 5721 IU

- **_Vitamin C:_** 13 milligrams

- **_Calcium:_** 114 milligrams

- **_Iron:_** 2 milligrams

Preparation time:
- Under 30 Minutes - This recipe takes under 30 minutes from start to finish

3. Beef Protein Bowl

A "Beef Protein Bowl" typically consists of beef as the main protein, served in a bowl with various accompaniments. Here's a general overview:

<u>*1. Beef:*</u> The primary ingredient and protein source, prepared in various ways like grilling, roasting, or stir-frying based on preference.

<u>*2. Vegetables:*</u> Typically includes a variety such as leafy greens (spinach, kale), tomatoes, cucumbers, bell peppers, or onions for flavor and nutrition.

<u>*3. Grains or Base:*</u> Often served over grains like brown rice, quinoa, or couscous, providing carbohydrates and fiber alongside the protein-rich beef.

4. Sauce or Dressing: A flavorful sauce or dressing adds moisture and enhances taste, ranging from tangy vinaigrettes to creamy tahini-based options.

5. Optional Additions: Additional toppings such as avocado, cheese, nuts, seeds, or herbs can be added for extra flavor, texture, or nutritional benefits.

A beef protein bowl is designed to offer a well-rounded, satisfying meal that combines protein, carbohydrates, healthy fats, and vegetables in one convenient dish. It's a popular choice for a nutritious and filling meal, often customizable to suit individual dietary preferences.

Protein, a crucial macronutrient essential for muscle development and satiety, plays a significant role in weight management and enhancing strength, supported by research.

For those managing migraine disorders, sufficient protein intake contributes to:

1. Maintaining stable blood sugar levels.
2. Reducing unhealthy snacking and promoting post-meal satisfaction.
3. Enhancing alertness and energy levels, especially during migraine episodes.

Comparing this beef protein bowl, providing 34 grams of protein along with plenty of vegetables, with other "protein bowl" recipes offering less than 12 grams emphasizes its high protein content and suitability for low-carb or keto diets. It's important to complement high-protein meals with complex carbohydrates, vegetables, and healthy fats to maintain a balanced diet.

ingredient list:
- 1 pound of ground beef
- Kosher salt and black pepper
- Olive oil
- 8 ounces of cauliflower rice
- 1/2 teaspoon of chili powder
- 1/2 teaspoon of cumin
- 1/2 teaspoon of smoked paprika
- 2 zucchini squash, cubed
- 1 cup of spinach
- 2 large eggs
- 2 green onions, chopped
- Salsa verde or any type of salsa

Preparation Time: 5 minutes
- Cooking Time: 20 minutes
- Total Time: 25 minutes
- Servings: 3 servings

- Calories: 485 kcal

Instructions:

1. Brown ground beef in a large non-stick pan over medium-high heat until fully cooked and crumbled, stirring regularly (about 5-6 minutes). Season with salt and pepper, then remove from the pan and set aside.

2. In the same pan, add a teaspoon of olive oil and cauliflower rice. Sprinkle it with chili powder, cumin, and smoked paprika. Sauté over medium heat for 1-2 minutes, then add zucchini and cook for another 2-3 minutes until slightly tender. Season with ¼ teaspoon of salt and a pinch of pepper. Set aside.

3. Clean the pan with a paper towel. Heat another teaspoon of olive oil over medium-high heat. Crack eggs into the pan, taking care not to break the yolks. Cook until the egg whites are

set, then flip and cook for another 20-40 seconds for over easy/medium eggs. Meanwhile, lightly wilt the spinach on the other side of the pan.

4. Combine the cauliflower rice mixture with zucchini in a bowl. Top with the cooked ground beef, eggs, and spinach. Adjust seasoning to taste and garnish with salsa and chopped green onions before serving.

Nutritional Information:
- Energy: 485 kilocalories
- Carbohydrates: 11 grams
- Protein: 34 grams
- Fat: 34 grams
- Saturated Fat: 13 grams
- Polyunsaturated Fat: 2 grams
- Monounsaturated Fat: 14 grams
- Trans Fat: 2 grams
- Cholesterol: 216 milligrams
- Sodium: 203 milligrams

- Potassium: 1227 milligrams
- Fiber: 4 grams
- Sugars: 6 grams
- Vitamin A: 1704 IU
- Vitamin C: 82 milligrams
- Calcium: 110 milligrams
- Iron: 5 milligrams

4. Grilled Italian Shrimp

"Grilled Italian Shrimp" refers to shrimp seasoned with Italian-inspired flavors, then grilled until fully cooked and slightly charred, offering a taste reminiscent of the Mediterranean. It's often served as a main dish or part of a seafood meal, accompanied by sides such as salad, pasta, or grilled vegetables.

Shrimp is a nutritious protein source rich in omega-3 fatty acids, zinc, and vitamin B12, supporting immune function and brain health. This recipe is suitable for various diets including the Heal Your Headache migraine diet, dairy-free, gluten-free, paleo, and whole30 (excluding honey). The marinade can be quickly prepared in a food processor without the need for chopping. Grilling simplifies cleanup, though a grill pan is a suitable alternative.

Ingredients

- 2 large garlic cloves, peeled
- 2 tablespoons fresh basil
- 1 tablespoon fresh parsley
- 1.5 teaspoon dried thyme
- 1 teaspoon honey
- 1 tablespoon tomato paste
- 3 tablespoons extra virgin olive oil
- 1.5 tablespoons distilled white vinegar
- ½ teaspoon kosher salt
- 1 pound peeled and deveined jumbo or extra large RAW shrimp, tail on fresh or frozen and defrosted is fine
- fresh black pepper to taste

- ***Preparation Time:*** 10 minutes

- ***Cooking Time:*** 5 minutes

- ***Marinating Time:*** 30 minutes

- ***Total Time:*** 45 minutes

- ***Servings:*** 3

- ***Calories:*** 293 kcal

Instructions:

1. If your shrimp isn't deveined, it's easy to prepare. Remove the shell, which is usually pre-cut, and use a small knife to make a slit along the back of each shrimp. You'll find a dark "line" exposed; remove it and rinse the shrimp. Pat them dry.

2. In a food processor, blend all ingredients except the shrimp until the mixture is almost smooth. Pour the sauce over the shrimp, toss to coat evenly, and refrigerate to marinate for 30 minutes to an hour. If you're planning to grill, thread the shrimp on skewers.

3. Preheat your grill or grill pan to medium-high heat. Place the shrimp on the hot grill or pan and cook without moving them for 2 minutes. Flip them over and cook for another 2-3 minutes on the other side, adjusting the time based on the size of your shrimp. The shrimp should become opaque throughout without any clear or grayish parts.

4. Serve the shrimp immediately or cover and refrigerate for up to 2 days.

Nutritional Information:

- ***Energy:*** 293 calories

- ***Carbs:*** 4 grams

- ***Protein:*** 31 grams

- ***Fat:*** 16 grams

- ***Saturated Fat:*** 2 grams

- ***Cholesterol:*** 381 milligrams

- ***Sodium:*** 1606 milligrams

- ***Potassium:*** 200 milligrams

- ***Fiber:*** 1 gram

- ***Sugar:*** 3 grams

- **_Vitamin A:_** 283 IU

- **_Vitamin C:_** 10 milligrams

- **_Calcium:_** 239 milligrams

- **_Iron:_** 4 milligrams

5. Chicken Zucchini Poppers with Creamy Cilantro Sauce

Chicken Zucchini Poppers with Creamy Cilantro Sauce are small, flavorful appetizers made from ground chicken, grated zucchini, and a blend of herbs and spices. Here's a breakdown of the dish:

1. Chicken Zucchini Poppers:

- **_Ingredients:_** Typically include ground chicken, grated zucchini, minced garlic, onion powder, paprika, salt, pepper, and sometimes egg and breadcrumbs for binding.

- **_Preparation:_** Mix ingredients to form small patties or balls, then pan-fry or bake until golden brown and fully cooked.

- **_Flavor Profile:_** Offers a juicy texture from chicken and zucchini, with savory and mildly spicy flavors from the seasonings.

2. Creamy Cilantro Sauce:

Creamy cilantro sauce is a versatile condiment that combines the vibrant taste of cilantro with a creamy foundation.

Ingredients

- 1 pound of ground chicken (at least 7% fat recommended)
- 1 to 2 medium zucchini squash, shredded (about 1½ cups)
- 2 cloves of garlic, minced
- 2 tablespoons of fresh chives, chopped
- ½ teaspoon of kosher salt
- ¼ teaspoon of freshly ground black pepper
- 1 to 2 tablespoons of oil for cooking

For the Creamy Cilantro Sauce:

- 1 cup of fresh cilantro
- 1 small garlic clove (adjust to taste)
- ⅓ cup of mayonnaise
- 1 tablespoon of cottage cheese
- 1 tablespoon of distilled white vinegar

Preparation time

- **Prep Time:** 15 minutes

- **Cook Time**: 8 minutes

- **Total Time:** 23 minutes

- **Servings:** 6 patties

- **Calories per serving:** 204 kcal

Instructions:
1. Mix cilantro, garlic, and cheese sauce in a blender.
2. Grate zucchini and remove excess water.
3. Mix chicken, garlic, and zucchini in a bowl.
4. Make 6 patties from the mixture.
5. Cook patties in a skillet for 4 minutes on each side.
6. Serve hot with dipping sauce."

Nutrition Facts (per serving of 2 patties):

- Energy: 204 calories
- Macronutrients:
-   Carbs: 2g
-   Protein: 14g
-   Fat: 16g
- Vitamins and Minerals:
-   Vitamin A: 289IU
-   Vitamin C: 7mg
-   Calcium: 15mg
-   Iron: 1mg
- Other nutrients:
-   Fiber: 1g
-   Sugar: 1g
-   Sodium: 331mg
-   Potassium: 494mg
-   Cholesterol: 71mg
-   Saturated Fat: 3g"

6.4 Quick Recovery smoothie

Quick Recovery smoothie" is likely a specific recipe aimed at helping individuals recover from vestibular migraine symptoms. Vestibular migraines cause vertigo, dizziness, and balance issues without typical headache pain.

This smoothie typically includes ingredients known for managing migraine symptoms and aiding recovery. While recipes vary, common components might be:

1. Ginger: Recognized for its anti-inflammatory and anti-nausea properties, ginger can ease nausea and potentially reduce migraine-related dizziness.

2. Leafy greens: Such as spinach or kale, rich in magnesium, which can relax blood vessels and potentially lessen migraine frequency.

3. Berries: Like blueberries, strawberries, or raspberries, rich in antioxidants that reduce oxidative stress and inflammation linked to migraines.

4. Greek yogurt or almond milk: Providing a creamy base and calcium and vitamin D, potentially aiding in migraine prevention.

5. Banana: High in potassium, regulating fluid balance and potentially easing symptoms like dizziness.

6. Flaxseeds or chia seeds: Containing omega-3 fatty acids that have anti-inflammatory properties, potentially reducing migraine intensity and frequency.

7. Honey or agave syrup: Occasionally added for sweetness, with caution due to sugar's potential migraine-triggering effects.

This smoothie is crafted to be easily digestible, packed with nutrients supporting recovery and symptom management during or after a vestibular migraine episode. It's crucial for those with vestibular migraines to discuss dietary approaches with healthcare providers to identify helpful or aggravating ingredients.

9. Anti-Inflammatory Smoothie

An anti-inflammatory smoothie usually consists of a blend of ingredients renowned for their anti-inflammatory properties. These ingredients commonly include:

1. Leafy greens: Examples include spinach, kale, or Swiss chard, known for their antioxidants and phytochemicals that combat inflammation.

2. Berries: Particularly blueberries, strawberries, or raspberries, which are rich in antioxidants like anthocyanins that have anti-inflammatory effects.

3. Turmeric: This spice contains curcumin, recognized for its potent anti-inflammatory properties.

4.Ginger: Another spice containing gingerol, which has demonstrated anti-inflammatory and pain-reducing properties.

5. Healthy fats: Such as avocado or flaxseed oil, providing omega-3 fatty acids that can help reduce inflammation.

6. Nuts and seeds: Examples include walnuts, chia seeds, or flaxseeds, which are high in omega-3s and antioxidants.

7.Green tea: Adding brewed green tea or matcha powder can offer additional antioxidants and anti-inflammatory compounds.

To prepare an anti-inflammatory smoothie, blend these ingredients with a liquid base like water, coconut water, almond milk, or dairy-free yogurt until smooth. This combination not only tastes great but also promotes overall health by reducing inflammation within the body.

Ingredients:

- ¾ cup pear (with skin)
- 2 teaspoons fresh ginger
- ¾ cup fresh spinach
- ¾ cup oat milk
- 2 teaspoons hemp or chia seeds
- 1 teaspoon honey or maple syrup (opt)

1. Anti-Inflammatory Smoothie Recipe:

This smoothie is a game-changer for inflammation and migraine relief. With pear, spinach, ginger, and chia seeds, it's packed with nutrients that fight pain and promote gut health. The Mediterranean diet inspired this recipe, which balances protein, fiber, and healthy fats.

<u>**Pear:**</u> Rich in antioxidants and fiber, pears promote heart health, weight loss, and gut health.

Ginger: Natural anti-inflammatory that aids in nausea and pain relief.

Greens: Boosts magnesium levels, which can help prevent migraine attacks.

Seeds: Hemp or chia seeds add protein and balance the sugar content.

This smoothie is easy on the stomach, migraine-friendly, and packed with omega-3s. Try it today and experience the benefits for yourself!"

"Recipe Details:
- Preparation Time: 10 minutes
- Cooking Time: 30 minutes
- Total Time: 40 minutes
- Servings: 4 people
- Calories per serving: 398 calories"

Instructions:

"Blend the following ingredients until smooth:

- Pear
- Ginger
- Spinach
- Milk
- Seeds

- Add ice (about ½ cup) and blend until the mixture is smooth and frothy. If desired, add a sweetener like honey or maple syrup to taste."

"Recipe Details:

- **Prep Time:** 10 minutes
- **Total Time:** 10 minutes
- Servings: 1 serving
- Calories per serving: 209 calories"

2. Gut-Boosting Post-Workout Smoothie

"Fuel your body after a workout with a Gut-Boosting Post-Workout Smoothie! This nutrient-packed drink supports gut health, muscle recovery, and overall well-being. It typically includes:

- Probiotics for a healthy gut microbiome
- Prebiotic fiber to feed good bacteria
- Protein for muscle repair
- Anti-inflammatory ingredients like turmeric or ginger
- Fiber-rich fruits and veggies like bananas, spinach, or kale

Example ingredients include probiotic yogurt, banana, spinach, protein powder, almond milk, chia seeds, and turmeric. This smoothie:

- Replenishes energy stores
- Supports muscle recovery
- Promotes gut health and digestion
- Reduces inflammation and oxidative stress

Indulge in a Gut-Boosting Post-Workout Smoothie after your next exercise session to support your overall health and wellness!"

Recipe Details:
- Preparation Time: 5 minutes
- Total Time: 5 minutes

Ingredients List:
- 2 cups of low-fat kefir (plain)

- 1 ripe banana
- 2 cups of frozen blueberries
- ½ of a ripe avocado
- A 1-inch piece of fresh ginger, peeled
- 2 tablespoons of chia seeds

Instructions:

1. Add all the ingredients to a blender and blend on high speed for about 1 minute, until the mixture is smooth and creamy.
2. Pour and serve immediately!

Nourishment Facts (per serving):

- Energy: 355 calories
- Fat: 13g (of which saturated fat: 2.8g)
- Protein: 15g
- Carbohydrates: 51g
- Fiber: 10.9g
- Sugar: 32.6g (naturally occurring, no added sugars)
- Sodium: 133 mg

3. Healthy Blueberry Smoothie

"This blueberry smoothie is a brain-boosting powerhouse! Here's why:

- Berry fruits like blueberries have been shown to protect brain health, improving cognitive function, motor skills, and neuroplasticity.

- Blueberries support gut health, promoting healthy digestion and regularity.

- This smoothie is a great low-histamine option for those with histamine intolerance.

- The high antioxidant content in blueberries makes them a popular ingredient in supplements that combat brain fog and memory loss, like magnesium threonate.

Recipe Details:
- Preparation Time: 5 minutes
- Total Time: 5 minutes
- Servings: 1 serving
- Calories per serving: 325 calories

Equipment Needed:
- 1 high-powered blender (such as Ninja, Nutribullet, or Vitamix)

Ingredients List:
- 1 cup of frozen wild blueberries
- 2 tablespoons of dried mulberries (a game-changer for flavor and nutrition)
- 2 tablespoons of creamy sunbutter
- A hint of vanilla extract (½ teaspoon)

- ¾ cup of your favorite milk
- Ice cubes (½ cup) to chill and thicken the mix

Blending Instructions:

1. Add blueberries, mulberries, sunbutter, vanilla, and milk to the blender.
2. Pulse to grind the mixture, then increase speed to blend until smooth.
3. Add any optional add-ins (like greens or seeds) with the initial ingredients.
4. Use a blender tamper to scrape down the sides and avoid adding excess liquid.

5. If desired, add approximately ½ cup of ice to thicken the mixture.

6. Blend until smooth and enjoy!"

"Nourishment Facts (per serving):

- Energy: 325 calories
- Carbs: 25g
- Protein: 10g
- Fat: 20g (with 2g saturated, 3g polyunsaturated, and 0.5g monounsaturated)
- Sodium: 109 mg
- Potassium: 278 mg
- Fiber: 6g
- Sugar: 17g
- Vitamins: 473 IU of Vitamin A, 26mg of Vitamin C
- Minerals: 281 mg of Calcium, 4mg of Iron

"Treat yourself to a glass of this delectable and nutritious Healthy Blueberry Smoothie, overflowing with cognitive benefits, digestive-friendly ingredients, and a wealth of antioxidants. Savor the creamy texture and sweet taste, and enjoy the perfect boost to start your day or energize your body anytime. Relish the flavor and reap the benefits of a healthier, happier you!"

Chapter 7: Dinner Delights

Chapter 7 of "Dinner Delights" begins in a charming village at dusk, filling the air with the inviting smells of homemade food and the gentle sounds of fine dining utensils. Within these pages, readers are immersed in a rich tapestry of flavors and familial closeness as the protagonist carefully prepares an extravagant dinner. From the sizzle of vegetables in a hot pan to the enticing aroma of sauces slowly simmering, every detail welcomes readers into a world where food symbolizes affection and heritage. Amid the gentle glow of candlelight and the laughter echoing through the room, Chapter 7 promises an experience that delights the senses, with each dish telling its own story of joy, introspection, and the simple pleasures found in sharing meals.

7.1 Flavorful and Nourishing Main Courses

This section features main dishes that not only satisfy the palate but also support well-being. From robust stews to light, nutritious meals, each recipe aims to blend flavors and nutrition seamlessly. Whether you need a quick weekday dinner or something to impress guests, these main courses promise satisfaction:

1. Fried Rice without Soy Sauce

"Create delicious fried rice without soy sauce by substituting it with other flavorful ingredients that pack an umami punch. Try using:

Preparation Recipe Details:
- Prep: 10min
- Cook: 10min
- Total: 20min

- Servings: 4
- Calories: 416/serving"

Recipe Ingredients:

- Oil (3-4 tbsp)
- Eggs (2) (optional)
- Garlic (2 cloves)
- Green onion (¾ cup)
- -Mixed veggies (¾ cup)
- Kale/cabbage mix (3 cups)
- Brown rice (2 cups)
- Coconut aminos (2 tbsp)
- Sesame oil (2 tsp)
- Sweet chili sauce (2 tsp)
- Kosher salt (1 tsp)
- Optional: Sriracha"

"Cooking Instructions:

1. Heat oil, cook eggs (if using), and set aside.

2. Cook garlic, green onion, and veggies in the same pan.
3. Add cruciferous greens and cook until softened.
4. Add rice and egg mixture, stirring to combine.
5. Cook until rice is crispy and warmed through.
6. Mix sauce ingredients and pour into rice mixture.
7. Serve warm with sriracha on the side.

Nutrition Facts:

- Calories: 416
- Macros: 78g carbs, 11g protein, 7g fat
- Fat: 2g sat, 2g poly, 3g mono, 0.01g trans
- Cholesterol: 82mg
- Sodium: 209 mg
- Potassium: 402mg
- Fiber: 4g
- Sugar: 2g

- Vitamins: 1181IU A, 40mg C
- Minerals: 62 mg calcium, 3mg iron"

2. Grilled Salmon with Citrus Glaze:

Grilled Salmon with Citrus Glaze is a mouthwatering dish that showcases:

- Perfectly grilled salmon filets
- A tangy and sweet citrus glaze made with a blend of:
- Fresh citrus juice (orange, lemon, or lime)
- Honey or maple syrup
- Soy sauce or tamari
- Garlic and ginger
- Herbs like thyme or rosemary

The glaze is brushed onto the salmon during the last few minutes of grilling, creating a caramelized, sticky crust that complements the rich flavor of the fish. This dish is often served with:

- Roasted vegetables
- Whole grains like quinoa or brown rice
- Steamed asparagus or broccoli
- A simple green salad
-

It's a healthy, flavorful option perfect for a summer barbecue or a quick weeknight dinner!"

Preparation Recipe Details:
- Prep: 50min
- Cook: 15min
- Total: 1hr 5min
- Servings: 4
- Calories: 393/serving"

Ingredients:
- 1 lb salmon (4 filets)
- ¾ cup brown sugar
- 1 orange

- 2 lemons
- 1 tsp kosher salt
- 1 tsp black pepper
- 2 tbsp butter (sliced)"

Instructions:

1. Zest the entire lemon, orange, and grapefruit and mix with brown sugar in a bowl.
2. Place a salmon filet on a large piece of foil sprayed with non-stick spray.
3. Season with salt and pepper, then rub the zest mixture evenly over the filet.
4. Place butter tabs on top of the filet.
5. Cover with slices of lemon, orange, and grapefruit.
6. Seal the foil pack and marinate at room temperature for 45 minutes.
7. Preheat the grill to hot, then reduce heat to warm except for one burner.

8. Cook salmon opposite the hot burner for 10-15 minutes, until opaque and flaky.

"Nutrition Facts (per filet):

- Calories: 393
- Macros: 47g carbs, 23g protein, 13g fat
- Fat: 4g sat, 77mg chol
- Sodium: 694mg
- Potassium: 707 mg
- Fiber: 1g
- Sugar: 43g
- Vitamins: 295 IU A, 31.8mg C
- Minerals: 68mg calcium, 1.4mg iron"

3. Baked Chicken Kabobs

"Baked Chicken Kabobs: A Delicious and Healthy Meal

Preparation Recipe Details:

- Prep: 10min
- Cook: 20min
- Marinate: 30min
- Total: 60min
- Servings: 4
- Calories: 294/serving"

Ingredients:
- Chicken pieces (breast or thighs)
- Colorful bell peppers
- Onions
- Mushrooms
- Cherry tomatoes
- Olives
- Garlic
- Herbs (thyme, rosemary)
- Lemon juice/zest
- Olive oil
- Salt and pepper

Instructions:

1. Begin by cutting the chicken into 1-inch pieces and set them aside.
2. Combine the marinade ingredients (olive oil, Dijon mustard, garlic, oregano, sumac, salt, and pepper) in a large bowl.
3. Add the chicken to the marinade, ensuring it's evenly coated. Cover the bowl and refrigerate for 30 minutes to 12 hours.
4. Preheat your oven to 425°F (220°C). Thread the marinated chicken, along with peppers and shallots, onto skewers.
5. Bake the skewers for 15-20 minutes until the chicken is fully cooked (no pink inside, with an internal temperature of 165°F as measured by a meat thermometer).
6. For a grilled-like charred finish, broil the kabobs about 6 inches from the heat source for 1-2 minutes until lightly charred.
7. Serve the kabobs warm and enjoy!

Note: Line a baking sheet with aluminum foil for easier cleanup."

"Nutrition Facts (per serving):

- Calories: 294
- Macros: 8g carbs, 38g protein, 12g fat
- Fat: 2g sat, 1g poly, 7g mono, 1g trans
- Cholesterol: 109 mg
- Sodium: 535mg
- Potassium: 840mg
- Fiber: 2g
- Sugar: 3g
- Vitamins: 1055 IU A, 97 mg C
- Minerals: 36mg calcium, 1 mg iron"

7.2 Comforting Side Dishes

Enhance your main course with these comforting sides that add texture and flavor diversity to your meal. From timeless classics to innovative creations, these dishes are designed to complement any dinner setting:

1. Garlic Parmesan Roasted Brussels Sprouts:

Brussels sprouts roasted until crispy and caramelized, then tossed with garlic, Parmesan cheese, and a hint of lemon zest.

"Recipe Timeline:

- Total Time: 50 minutes
- Preparation Time: 10 minutes
- Cooking Time: 40 minutes"

Ingredients:

- 1 lb Brussels sprouts, halved
- 4 tbsp olive oil
- ½ tsp salt
- 1 tsp pepper
- 1 tsp garlic powder
- ¼ cup bread crumbs
- ¼ cup grated parmesan cheese

Instructions:

1. Prepare Brussels sprouts by removing stems and halving them.
2. Place sprouts in a large bowl and add remaining ingredients.
3. Toss to coat sprouts evenly.
4. Spread sprouts on a baking sheet.
5. Bake in a preheated 400°F (200°C) oven for 20 minutes.
6. Flip sprouts and continue baking for an additional 20 minutes or until tender and golden.
7. Enjoy your delicious roasted Brussels sprouts!

Tips:

- Don't overcook, check for tenderness.
- Add extra parmesan cheese for flavor.
- Use freshly grated parmesan rind for extra flavor.
- Add minced garlic for extra flavor.
- Use shake n bake instead of bread crumbs for a different texture.
- Adjust cooking time based on your oven.

Enjoy your delicious roasted Brussels sprouts!"

2. Herbed Quinoa Pilaf

Herbed Quinoa Pilaf: Nutty quinoa is cooked with a blend of fresh herbs to create a light and fluffy pilaf that pairs beautifully with any main dish.

Ingredients:
- 1 cup quinoa
- 2 cups water or broth
- 2 tbsp olive oil
- 1 small onion, chopped
- 2 cloves garlic, minced
- 1 cup mixed fresh herbs (parsley, basil, thyme, rosemary)
- Salt and pepper to taste
- Optional: lemon zest and juice

Prep Time: 15 minutes

Instructions:

1. Rinse quinoa and cook in water or broth for 15-20 minutes.
2. Heat olive oil in a skillet and sauté onion and garlic until softened.
3. Add fresh herbs, salt, and pepper to the skillet and stir to combine.
4. Fluff cooked quinoa with a fork and added it to the skillet. Stir to combine.
5. If using lemon zest and juice, stir them in at this point.
6. Serve hot and enjoy!

Nutrition Facts (per serving):

- Calories: 350
- Protein: 8g
- Fat: 10g
- Saturated Fat: 1.5g

- Carbohydrates: 50g
- Fiber: 5g
- Sugar: 2g
- Sodium: 200mg
- Potassium: 400mg
- Vitamin A: 10% DV
- Vitamin C: 20% DV
- Calcium: 5% DV
- Iron: 15% DV

"Note: Nutritional values are estimated and could differ depending on ingredients used and serving sizes."

"In essence, Herbed Quinoa Pilaf is a tasty and nourishing dish that blends quinoa's earthy flavor with the freshness of herbs. It's a flexible and simple recipe ideal for a wholesome lunch or dinner. Packed with protein and fiber, this pilaf is a great choice for a satisfying and nutritious meal. The addition of lemon zest and juice provides a refreshing citrusy taste that complements the herbs wonderfully. Whether you're vegetarian, vegan, or just looking for a nutritious and flavorful meal, Herbed Quinoa Pilaf is an excellent option. Try it out to enjoy its delicious flavors and health benefits!"

3.Creamy Mashed Sweet Potatoes:

"Indulge in the comfort of Creamy Mashed Sweet Potatoes, a delectable side dish crafted from tender sweet potatoes, blended with a medley of ingredients to achieve a velvety smoothness. The recipe features:

"Ingredients:

- 3 pounds (1360g) sweet potatoes, cleaned and peeled (about 5-6 medium-sized potatoes)
- 1 ½ teaspoons fine sea salt, with extra for seasoning
- 1 bay leaf
- 3 tablespoons butter
- 1/8 teaspoon ground cinnamon

- 3 tablespoons sour cream or heavy cream (optional)

Optional toppings:
- Finely chopped parsley or chives
- Freshly ground black pepper

- Note: You'll need 5-6 medium sweet potatoes, which equal approximately 3 pounds or 1360g."

Instructions:

1. Peel and cube sweet potatoes into 1-inch pieces.
2. Boil them in a large pot with enough water to cover, adding salt and a bay leaf. Simmer for 10-12 minutes until tender.

3. Drain and mash the sweet potatoes in the pot or use a food processor to achieve your desired consistency.

4. Add butter, cinnamon, black pepper, and a pinch of salt. For an extra creamy texture, stir in sour cream or heavy cream.

5. Serve and enjoy!"

"Nutrition Facts (per serving):

- Serving size: approximately 3/4 cup
- Calories: 257
- Fat: 6.7g (with 4.2g saturated)
- Cholesterol: 17.4mg
- Sodium: 711.1mg
- Carbohydrates: 46.2g
- Fiber: 6.9g
- Sugars: 9.5g
- Protein: 4.1g

Creamy Mashed Sweet Potatoes are a beloved side dish, especially during holidays, offering a delightful way to savor the natural sweetness of sweet potatoes in a rich and comforting way."

7.3 One-Pot Meals for Easy Cooking

Ideal for busy nights, these one-pot wonders simplify cooking while delivering robust flavors. These recipes minimize cleanup and maximize taste, making them perfect for hectic schedules:

1. Spicy Sausage and Vegetable Skillet:
"Prepare a quick and vibrant skillet dinner in just 30 minutes, featuring sausage, bell peppers, zucchini, corn, and fresh cilantro. This easy one-pan meal is ideal for meal prep and busy weeknights, making it a perfect solution for families on-the-go!"

Which variety of pre-cooked sausage is recommended?

For this recipe, select a pre-cooked sausage that is already seasoned with robust flavors. Great choices include smoked sausage, andouille sausage, or Cajun sausage. Italian sausage links are also suitable—whether sweet, mild, or spicy—provided they are fully cooked. Alternatively, crumbled sausage is another option; just make sure it's well-cooked before adding it to the skillet.

"Recipe Details:

- Preparation time: 15 minutes
- Cooking time: 15 minutes
- Total time: 30 minutes
- Servings: 4 people
- Calories per serving: 370 kcal
- Course: Main Course
- Cuisine: American"

"Recipe Ingredients:

- 2 cups cooked corn kernels (from 3 ears)

- 1 tablespoon olive oil
- 12 oz pre-cooked sausage (such as Cajun, andouille, or smoked)
- 1 large red bell pepper, diced
- 1 large zucchini, sliced
- ½ teaspoon chili powder
- Chopped fresh cilantro"

Instructions:

1. Cook sliced sausage in a cast-iron skillet with olive oil over medium heat, flipping halfway through. Remove and set aside.
2. Cook diced bell pepper and sliced zucchini in the same skillet, adding reserved oil as needed. Remove and set aside with sausage.
3. Add corn kernels to the skillet and cook briefly.
4. Combine cooked sausage, veggies, and corn in the skillet. Mix well, adding reserved oil and chili powder. Reheat on low heat.

5. Top with chopped cilantro and serve. (Salt may not be necessary due to the sausage's natural saltiness, but season to taste if desired.)

Nutritional Information:

- Spicy Sausage and Vegetable Skillet Nutrition Facts (per serving, assumes 4 servings)

- Calories: 370
- Macronutrients:
- Protein: 26g
- Fat: 24g (8g saturated)
- Carbohydrates: 20g (4g fiber, 6g sugar)
- Sodium: 450mg
- Cholesterol: 60mg
- Vitamins and Minerals:
- Vitamin A: 20% of the Daily Value (DV)
- Vitamin C: 40% of the DV
- Calcium: 10% of the DV
- Iron: 20% of the DV

- Potassium: 25% of the DV

Breakdown by Ingredient
- Sausage (12 oz): 240 calories, 16g protein, 16g fat, 400mg sodium
- Bell pepper (1 large): 49 calories, 1g protein, 0g fat, 10 mg sodium
- Zucchini (1 large): 25 calories, 1g protein, 0g fat, 10 mg sodium
- Corn kernels (1 cup): 80 calories, 2g protein, 1g fat, 10 mg sodium
- Olive oil (1 tbsp): 120 calories, 0g protein, 14g fat, 0mg sodium
- Chili powder and cilantro: negligible calories and nutrients

Note: Total values are approximate and may vary based on specific ingredients and portion sizes.

2. Coconut Curry Chicken and Rice

"Coconut Curry Chicken and Rice is a mouthwatering dish that blends the richness of coconut, the warmth of curry, and the savory flavors of chicken and rice. To make it, you'll need:

Prep Time: 5 minutes
Cooking Time: 25 minutes
Total Time: 30 minutes"

Ingredients list:
- Olive oil (2 tablespoons)
- Chicken breasts (2 pounds, cut into bite-sized pieces)
- Salt and pepper (to taste)
- Onion (1 small, chopped)
- Garlic (3 cloves, minced)
- Curry powder (2 tablespoons)
- Low-sodium chicken broth (1 cup)
- Coconut milk (1 can, 14 ounces)
- Diced tomatoes (1 can, 14.5 ounces)
- Tomato paste (2 tablespoons)

- Sugar (2 tablespoons)
- Fresh parsley (2 tablespoons, chopped)

Instructions:

1. Cook the chicken: Heat oil in a large skillet or Dutch oven. Add the chicken and season with salt and pepper. Cook for 5 minutes or until no longer pink.

2. Finish the dish: Add onion, garlic, curry powder, and cook for 2 minutes. Then add chicken broth, coconut milk, tomatoes, tomato paste, and sugar. Stir, bring to a boil, cover, and simmer for 15-20 minutes.

3. Garnish and serve: Sprinkle with parsley and serve over rice."

"Nutrition Facts (per serving):

- Energy: 396 calories (20% of daily need)

- Carbs: 13g (4% of daily need)
- Protein: 35g (70% of daily need)
- Fat: 23g (35% of daily need)
- Saturated Fat: 14g (88% of daily need)
- Cholesterol: 97 mg (32% of daily need)
- Sodium: 532mg (23% of daily need)
- Potassium: 977 mg (28% of daily need)
- Fiber: 2g (8% of daily need)
- Sugar: 7g (8% of daily need)
- Vitamin A: 5% of daily need
- Vitamin C: 15% of daily need
- Calcium: 6% of daily need
- Iron: 22% of daily need

In summary, Coconut Curry Chicken and Rice is a delightful culinary experience that seamlessly blends flavor and nutritional benefits. The harmonious mix of coconut milk, curry spices, chicken, and rice delivers a well-rounded array of essential nutrients, offering both satisfaction and healthiness. The inclusion of potassium and fiber from coconut milk and rice enriches the nutritional value of the dish. Whether you seek a swift dinner solution or a gourmet indulgence, this recipe promises to delight your palate while ensuring you feel both nourished and fulfilled.

3. Beef and Mushroom Stroganoff

Beef and Mushroom Stroganoff is a popular Russian-inspired dish made with sautéed beef, mushrooms, and a creamy sauce, typically served over egg noodles. Here's a breakdown of the dish:

- **Prep Time:** 10 minutes
- **Cook Time:** 30 minutes
- **Total Time:** 40 minutes
- **Servings:** 6 people

Ingredients list:
- 1 pound of egg fettuccine
- 4 tablespoons of butter
- 1 chopped onion

- 4 cloves of garlic, crushed or minced
- 1 pound of sliced mushrooms
- 24 ounces of lean beef filet, cut into 1 ½-inch cubes (sirloin, tenderloin, eye filet, or scotch filet)
- 2 teaspoons of Dijon mustard
- 1 teaspoon of paprika (smoky or mild)
- ⅓ cup of dry white wine (or more to taste)
- 2 cups of beef broth or stock (or 2 cups of water with 1 tablespoon of vegetable stock powder)
- 2 tablespoons of flour
- 1 tablespoon of Worcestershire sauce
- Salt and pepper to taste
- 1 cup of light sour cream (or reduced-fat cooking cream) at room temperature
- Fresh parsley, chopped (for garnish)"

Instructions

1. Cook pasta according to package directions until al dente, then drain and set aside.

2. Melt 2 tablespoons of butter in a large frying pan over medium heat. Cook steak in batches until browned, then set aside on a plate.

3. Melt remaining butter in the same pan. Add onions and cook until translucent, then add garlic and cook for 30 seconds.

4. Add mushrooms and cook until tender, about 4 minutes.

5. Add mustard, paprika, and wine to the pan, stirring to deglaze and scrape up browned bits. Reduce wine by half, about 3 minutes.

6. Whisk together beef broth, flour, and Worcestershire sauce in a small bowl. Add to the pan and simmer for 5 minutes, stirring occasionally, until sauce thickens.

7. Return beef to the pan, add accumulated juices, and season with salt and pepper if desired. Reduce heat to low, stir in sour cream, and heat until hot but not boiling.

8. Add cooked pasta to the pan, garnish with parsley, and serve!

Nourishment Facts:
- Energy: 619 calories
- Macronutrients:
- Carbs: 65g
- Protein: 41g
- Fat: 21g
- Fat Breakdown:
- Saturated: 10g
- Polyunsaturated: 2g
- Monounsaturated: 6g
- Trans: 0.4g
- Cholesterol: 166 mg
- Sodium: 537mg
- Potassium: 1.02mg

- Fiber: 4g
- Sugar: 4g
- Vitamins:
- A: 588IU
- C: 5mg
- Minerals:
- Calcium: 136mg
- Iron: 4mg

Chapter 7 of our cookbook is designed to bring joy to your table with delicious flavors, wholesome ingredients, and practical cooking techniques. Whether you're cooking for family dinners or entertaining guests, these dinner delights are sure to impress and satisfy. Enjoy exploring new flavors and the rewarding experience of sharing great meals with loved ones!

Chapter 8: Snacks and Treats

Enter a world of delectable flavors and tempting treats with Chapter 6. This section delves into a variety of snacks crafted to satisfy every craving. Whether you crave the satisfying crunch of chips, the creamy smoothness of dips, or the indulgent sweetness of desserts, you'll find a collection of recipes that are easy to make yet irresistibly delicious. Expand your snack options with creative ideas suitable for any occasion. Chapter 6 invites you to embark on a culinary journey where each snack time promises pure enjoyment.

8.1 Healthy Snack Options

Discover a variety of nutritious snack alternatives that satisfy cravings without sacrificing health. This section includes fresh fruit combinations, crunchy veggie sticks paired with tasty dips, and other guilt-free snacking ideas.

Sample Recipes:

1. Seasonal Fruit Salad

A Seasonal Fruit Salad is a delightful and refreshing dessert or snack comprising a variety of fruits that are currently in season. It usually includes:

1. Fresh berries such as strawberries, blueberries, raspberries, and blackberries.
2. Citrus fruits like oranges, grapefruits, and lemons.
3. Stone fruits include peaches, nectarines, plums, and cherries.
4. Tropical fruits include pineapple, mango, kiwi, and papaya.
5. Apples and pears, particularly in the fall and winter months.

To prepare, the fruits are typically washed, sliced, or chopped, and combined in a bowl. The salad is served either chilled or at room temperature. For added flavor, a splash of citrus juice like lemon or lime, and a touch of sugar or honey can be incorporated according to taste.

The versatility of a Seasonal Fruit Salad allows for creative adjustments based on personal preferences and the freshest fruits available during the current season.

Preparation Time: 20 minutes

Ingredients:

- 1 cup fresh strawberries, hulled and sliced
- 1 cup fresh blueberries
- 1 cup fresh grapes, halved
- 1 cup fresh pineapple, chunks
- 1 orange, peeled and segmented
- 1 apple, diced
- 2 tablespoons honey
- 1 tablespoon fresh lime juice
- Sprinkle of fresh mint leaves (optional)

Instructions:

1. In a large bowl, combine the sliced strawberries, blueberries, grapes, pineapple, and orange segments.
2. In a small bowl, whisk together the honey and lime juice until well combined.
3. Pour the honey-lime dressing over the fruit and toss to coat.
4. Add the diced apple and toss again.
5. Sprinkle with fresh mint leaves, if desired.
6. Serve immediately, or cover and refrigerate for up to 2 hours before serving.

Nutritional Information (per serving):

- Calories: 120
- Total Fat: 0.5g
- Saturated Fat: 0g
- Cholesterol: 0mg
- Sodium: 10mg
- Total Carbohydrates: 30g
- Dietary Fiber: 4g

- Sugars: 20g
- Protein: 1g
- Vitamin A: 10% DV
- Vitamin C: 100% DV
- Calcium: 2% DV
- Iron: 5% DV

Servings: 6-8

Note: Nutritional information is an estimate and may vary based on specific ingredients and portion sizes.

2. Greek Yogurt Parfait

"Indulge in a quick and easy breakfast or snack with this Greek Yogurt Parfait recipe. Layer Greek yogurt, fresh berries, and crunchy granola for a nutritious and delicious treat. Perfect for meal prep or a 5-minute assembly, this parfait is a great way to start your day. If you enjoy healthy yogurt desserts, also check out my recipes for Yogurt Fruit Dip and Chia Yogurt Pudding. Enjoy!"

Yields: 1 servings

Prep Time: 10 minutes mins

Total Time: 10 minutes mins

Ingredients

1. Optional sweetener: 1 tablespoon of honey or maple syrup (for drizzling)
2. Base: ¾ cup (180ml) of plain Greek yogurt
3. Fresh addition: ¼ cup (30g) of mixed berries (or other fruits) cut into 1-inch (2.5cm) pieces
4. Crunchy topping: ¼ cup (30g) of homemade or store-bought granola

Instructions:

1. Mix sweetener (1 tablespoon) with Greek yogurt (¾ cup) in a small bowl until fully incorporated.

2. Build the parfait in a jar or bowl:

- **_Layer 1:_** Add half of the yogurt mix (90ml)

- **_Layer 2:_** Add half of the fruit (15g)

- **_Layer 3:_** Sprinkle with half of the granola (15g)

3. Repeat the layers:

- **_Layer 4:_** Add the remaining yogurt mix (90ml)

- **_Layer 5:_** Add the remaining fruit (15g)

- **_Layer 6:_** Sprinkle with the remaining granola (15g)

4. Optional: Drizzle with an extra tablespoon of honey for added sweetness.

5. Serve and enjoy your delicious yogurt parfait!

Nutrition Information:
- 298 calories
- 28g of carbohydrates
- 21g of protein
- 11g of fat (including 3g of saturated fat, 2g of polyunsaturated fat, and 3g of monounsaturated fat)
- 10mg of cholesterol
- 78 mg of sodium
- 185 mg of potassium
- 4g of fiber
- 16g of sugar
- 122 IU of Vitamin A
- 1 mg of Vitamin C
- 225mg of Calcium
- 1 mg of Iron

This nutritious snack is a great way to support your overall health and well-being!"

3. Hummus with Veggie Sticks

Hummus with veggie sticks is a popular and nutritious snack or appetizer. Here's what it typically includes:

1. Hummus: A creamy dip made from mashed chickpeas, blended with tahini, olive oil, lemon juice, garlic, and salt, offering a smooth texture with a subtle nutty taste.

2. Veggie Sticks: Raw vegetables like carrots, cucumbers, bell peppers, celery, and cherry tomatoes, cut into stick shapes for easy dipping into hummus.

Preparation and Serving:

1. Hummus: Can be store-bought or homemade by blending chickpeas, tahini, olive oil, lemon juice, garlic, and salt until smooth. Adjust ingredients to taste.

2. Veggie Sticks: Wash and cut vegetables into sticks or slices, arranging them around a bowl of hummus for serving.

Nutritional Benefits:

1. Hummus: High in protein, fiber, and healthy fats from chickpeas and olive oil. It also provides essential vitamins and minerals, especially if prepared with fresh lemon juice and garlic.

2. Veggies: Low in calories and rich in vitamins, minerals, and fiber, adding crunch and freshness to complement the hummus.

Enjoying Hummus with Veggie Sticks:

- Dip veggie sticks into hummus for a nutritious snack or appetizer.

- Provides a balanced mix of protein, healthy fats, and micronutrients.

Variations:

1.Flavored Hummus: Experiment with flavors like roasted red pepper, spinach, or spicy hummus for added variety.

2.Veggie Options: Use different vegetables based on personal preference or seasonal availability.

Hummus with veggie sticks offers both delicious flavor and a healthy way to include more vegetables in your diet, making it a satisfying and nutritious choice for snacking.

8.2 Indulgent Treats with a Purpose:

Indulge in treats that are both delicious and nutritious. Recipes in this section feature dark chocolate truffles infused with antioxidants, fiber-rich oatmeal cookies, and homemade nut butter cups enhanced with sea salt.

Sample Recipes:

1. Dark Chocolate Avocado Truffles

Dark Chocolate Avocado Truffles are a luxurious dessert that combines the richness of dark chocolate with the smooth texture of avocado. Here's how they're made:

"How to prepare avocado chocolate truffles."

"Melt chocolate chips by:

1. Heat water in a saucepan until simmering.
2. Place a heat-safe bowl with chocolate chips over the pot.
3. Stirring until melted.
Or, melt in the microwave in 30-second increments, stirring between each interval."

"Chill the chocolate mixture in the fridge for 20 minutes. Then:

4. Scoop out small balls using a tablespoon or cookie scoop.
5. Roll them into smooth balls by hand.
6. Roll the balls in cocoa powder, nuts, or coconut flakes (if desired).
7. Enjoy immediately or store in an airtight container in the fridge for up to 1 week or freeze for up to 6 months."

What makes truffles so creamy?

"Truffles are notoriously creamy due to the traditional use of heavy cream. However, avocados can provide a similar creamy texture without the need for dairy, thanks to their healthy fats. This makes avocados an excellent substitute for heavy cream in truffle recipes."

Recipe Overview:

- **Preparation time:** 10 minutes
- **Cooking time:** 0 minutes (no cooking required)
- **Chilling time:** 20 minutes
- **Total time:** 30 minutes
- **Yield:** 15 servings"

"Ingredients:

- Chocolate chips (6 ounces / 1 cup): dark or semi-sweet

- Mashed avocado (⅓ cup): tightly packed

- Vanilla extract (½ teaspoon)

- Salt (a pinch)

- Cocoa powder (2 tablespoons): optional for rolling

Instructions:

1. Melt the chocolate chips using a microwave or a heat-safe bowl over simmering water.
2. In a separate bowl, mash the avocado until smooth and measure out ⅓ cup.
3. Combine the mashed avocado, vanilla extract, and salt in a large bowl.
4. Add the melted chocolate and mix until well combined and no avocado lumps remain.

5. Chill the mixture in the fridge for 20 minutes.

6. Scoop out 15 balls of chocolate and roll them between your palms to shape into smooth truffles.

7. Optional: roll the truffles in cocoa powder, shredded coconut, or crushed nuts for coating.

8. Serve immediately or store in an airtight container in the fridge. For a softer texture, let them come to room temperature before serving."

"Nutrition Facts:

- Energy: 64 calories
- Macronutrients:
- Carbohydrates: 8g
- Protein: 1g
- Fat: 3g
- Fat Breakdown:
- Saturated: 2g
- Polyunsaturated: 0.1g

- Monounsaturated: 0.4g
- Trans: 0.02g
- Cholesterol: 2mg
- Sodium: 8mg
- Potassium: 26mg
- Fiber: 1g
- Sugar: 7g
- Vitamins:
- A: 30IU
- C: 0.4mg
- Minerals:
- Calcium: 14mg
- Iron: 0.3mg"

2. Oatmeal Raisin Cookies

Oatmeal raisin cookies are cookies created mainly from oats, raisins, flour, butter, eggs, and sugar. Known for their chewy texture, robust oat taste, and the natural sweetness of raisins, they often incorporate cinnamon and vanilla extract to enhance their flavor. These cookies are beloved for their comforting flavor profile and are commonly savored as a snack or treat.

"Recipe Time:

- **_Preparation:_** 45 minutes
- **_Cooking:_** 13 minutes
- **_Total:_** 1 hour
- **_Output:_** 26-30 cookies"

"Ingredients:

- 1 cup (16 Tbsp; 226g) unsalted butter, softened

- 1 cup (200g) brown sugar (light or dark)

- 1/4 cup (50g) granulated sugar

- 2 large eggs

- 1 Tbsp pure vanilla extract

- 1 Tbsp (15ml) unsulphured or dark molasses (not blackstrap)

- 1 1/2 cups (188g) all-purpose flour (spooned and leveled)

- 1 tsp baking soda

- 1 1/2 tsp ground cinnamon

- 1/2 tsp salt

- 3 cups (255g) old-fashioned whole rolled oats

- 1 cup (140g) raisins (optional)

- 1/2 cup (64g) chopped toasted walnuts (optional)

Note: Please see the recipe notes for specific instructions on the raisins."

Instructions:

1. Cream butter and sugar together using a mixer until smooth (2 minutes).
2. Add eggs and mix until combined (1 minute).
3. Scrape down the bowl as needed, then add vanilla and molasses and mix until combined.
4. In a separate bowl, whisk together flour, baking soda, cinnamon, and salt.
5. Add dry ingredients to wet ingredients and mix until combined.
6. Beat in oats, raisins, and walnuts (if using) on low speed.
7. Chill dough for 30-60 minutes or up to 2 days.
8. Preheat the oven to 350°F (177°C) and line baking sheets with parchment paper.
9. Roll dough into balls (about 2 tablespoons each) and place 2 inches apart on baking sheets.
10. Bake for 12-14 minutes or until lightly browned on the sides.

11. Let cool on a baking sheet for 5 minutes, then transfer to a wire rack to cool completely.

Note: The cookies will continue to sit on the baking sheet during the cooling process."

Nutritional information:
- Energy: 120-140 calories
- Macronutrients:
- Carbs: 25-30g
- Protein: 2-3g
- Fat: 4-5g
- Fiber: 2-3g (1-2g soluble, 1-2g insoluble)
- Sugars: 8-10g (4-5g added)
- Sodium: 50-60mg
- Cholesterol: 10-15mg
- Vitamins:
- A: 0-1% DV
- C: 0-1% DV
- Calcium: 2-3% DV
- Iron: 4-5% DV
- Other nutrients:

- Potassium: 4-5% DV
- Manganese: 10-15% DV
- Copper: 5-6% DV

Note: ***These values are estimates and may vary based on specific ingredients and portion sizes."***

3. Nut Butter Cups

Nut butter cups are a delightful confection that combines the rich flavors of nut butter and chocolate into a delicious treat. Here's a step-by-step guide on how to make them:

"Instructions to make Almond Butter Cups:

1. Prepare a muffin tin by lining it with 12 paper cups.
2. Melt chocolate and coconut oil in a microwave-safe bowl.
3. Chill almond butter in the freezer for 5-10 minutes to make it easier to handle.
4. Fill each muffin tin with a tablespoon of melted chocolate.
5. Gently tap the tray to remove any air bubbles.
6. Refrigerate for 5 minutes or until the chocolate is fully hardened."

"Next steps to complete the Almond Butter Cups:

6. Add a dollop of almond butter to the center of each muffin cup.
7. Gently flatten the almond butter slightly with your finger.
8. Cover the almond butter with an additional 1 1/2 tablespoons of melted chocolate.
9. Sprinkle a pinch of salt on top of each cup.

10. Refrigerate for 10 minutes to set the chocolate and serve."

"Customize your Almond Butter Cups with these flavor variations:

- Add a touch of sweetness with maple syrup, vanilla extract, or cinnamon for a seasonal twist.

- Experiment with different nut butters, such as peanut butter, cashew butter, or hazelnut butter, to change up the flavor profile.

- Switch up the chocolate by using dark chocolate chips for a richer taste or milk chocolate chips for a sweeter treat."

"Storage Tips for Almond Butter Cups:

- Due to their sensitive nature, keep them refrigerated until consumption to prevent melting.

- Short-term storage: Store in airtight containers in the refrigerator for several weeks.

- Long-term storage: Place in a freezer-safe container and store in the freezer for up to 3 months."

"Recipe Overview:

- **Preparation Time:** 15 minutes
- **Total Time:** 15 minutes
- **Yield:** 12 servings"

"Ingredients:

- **Chocolate chips:** 14 ounces (397g)
- **Coconut oil:** 2 tablespoons (30ml)
- **Almond butter:** 1/2 cup (120g)

- ***Flakey sea salt*** (optional)

Instructions:

1. Line a muffin tin with paper cups.
2. Melt chocolate and coconut oil together in a microwave-safe bowl or over a double boiler.
3. Chill almond butter in the freezer for 5-10 minutes to firm up.
4. Fill each muffin tin with 1 tablespoon of melted chocolate and tap gently to remove air bubbles.
5. Chill in the fridge for 5 minutes.
6. Add a dollop (about 2 teaspoons) of almond butter to the center of each cup.
7. Flatten slightly with your finger, keeping it away from the edges.
8. Cover with 1 1/2 tablespoons of melted chocolate and tap gently to flatten.
9. Sprinkle with flaky sea salt (optional).

"Nutrition Facts (per serving):
- Energy: 250 calories
- Macronutrients:
- Carbohydrates: 25g
- Protein: 4g
- Fat: 16g (including 7g saturated fat)
- Cholesterol: 5mg
- Sodium: 23 mg
- Potassium: 78mg
- Fiber: 2g
- Sugar: 21g
- Vitamins:
- Vitamin A: 74 IU
- Vitamin C: 1mg
- Minerals:
- Calcium: 75mg
- Iron: 1mg

Note: *These values are approximate and may vary based on specific ingredients and portion sizes."*

8.3 Homemade Energy Bars and Bites

Keep your energy levels up with homemade bars and bites perfect for a quick snack or post-workout boost. Customize these recipes with nuts, seeds, and dried fruits to suit your taste preferences and dietary needs.

Sample Recipes

1. No-Bake Nutty Energy Bars

"These homemade granola bars achieve a delightful blend of salty and sweet tastes. They're crafted by mixing assorted nuts, coconut, smooth almond butter, and honey for a delectable snack that's both nutritious and irresistible. Below are the essential ingredients for preparing these tasty granola bars:"

ingredients:

1.Start with 2 cups of assorted chopped nuts like almonds, pecans, and walnuts.

2.Add 1/2 cup of shredded coconut for sweetness and flavor.

3.Include 1/2 cup of raisins or another dried fruit for extra sweetness.

4.Sprinkle in a pinch of salt (about 1/4 tsp) for a savory touch.

5.Mix in 1/2 tsp of cinnamon for enhanced flavor.

6.Lastly, add 1/2 cup of almond butter to bind everything together and increase protein content.

These ingredients will come together to create a delicious and nutritious granola bar!"

"Recipe Timeline:

- **Preparation time:** 10 minutes

- **Cooking time:** 30 minutes

- **Total time:** 40 minutes

"Equipment Needed:
- Large mixing bowl
- Small mixing bowl
- Stirring utensil

- Loaf or brownie pan (size determines bar thickness)
- Spatula or pressing tool
- Measuring cups: 1/4 tsp, 1/2 tsp, 1 tsp, 1/4 cup, 1/2 cup, and 1 cup

Instructions:

1. In a large bowl, mix together the dry ingredients: nuts, coconut, raisins, salt, and cinnamon.

2. In a smaller bowl, combine the wet ingredients: almond butter, honey, coconut oil, and vanilla.

3. Add the wet ingredients to the dry ingredients and stir thoroughly until fully mixed.

4. Press the mixture firmly into a loaf or brownie pan.

5. Place the pan in the freezer and let it freeze for at least 2 hours.

6. Once frozen, remove from the freezer and cut into desired sizes.

Nutty Energy Bars:

Per serving (1 bar):
- Calories: 250-270
- Protein: 8-10g
- Fat: 12-14g
- Carbohydrates: 25-30g
- Fiber: 4-5g
- Sugar: 8-10g
- Sodium: 50-100mg
- Potassium: 200-250mg
- Vitamin A: 10-15% of the Daily Value (DV)
- Vitamin C: 5-10% of the DV
- Calcium: 10-15% of the DV
- Iron: 15-20% of the DV

Please note that this is an estimate and actual values may vary based on the specific ingredients and their measurements used in the recipe.

Enjoy your no-bake nutty granola bars!"

2. Chia Seed Energy Bites

Chia seed energy bites are nutritious snacks primarily made from chia seeds, alongside ingredients like nuts, dried fruits, honey or maple syrup, and sometimes oats or coconut flakes. Here's a breakdown of their components and advantages:

1. Chia Seeds: These tiny seeds are packed with nutrients like fiber, protein, omega-3 fatty acids, vitamins, and minerals. They are well-known for their capacity to soak up liquid and create a gel-like texture, which helps bind the ingredients together in energy bites.

2. Nuts: Commonly used varieties include almonds, walnuts, or cashews, adding healthy fats, protein, and a crunchy texture to the energy bites.

3.Dried Fruits: Examples include dates, apricots, raisins, or cranberries, contributing natural sweetness, fiber, and additional vitamins and minerals.

4.Natural Sweeteners: Honey, maple syrup, or agave syrup are frequently used to sweeten the bites naturally and aid in binding the ingredients.

5.Additional Ingredients: Depending on the recipe, ingredients such as oats, coconut flakes, cocoa powder, or nut butter may be included for flavor, texture, and nutritional benefits.

Benefits of Chia Seed Energy Bites:

1. Nutrient-Dense: They offer a concentrated source of nutrients including protein, healthy fats, fiber, vitamins, and minerals.

2. Sustained Energy: The blend of complex carbohydrates, protein, and healthy fats provides sustained energy, making them ideal snacks before or after workouts.

3. Fiber Content: Chia seeds, oats, and nuts are high in fiber, promoting digestion and satiety.

4. Antioxidants: Dried fruits and nuts contain antioxidants that combat inflammation and protect cells from damage.

5. Versatility: Recipes can be adjusted to suit various dietary preferences such as vegan or gluten-free diets.

Chia seed energy bites are straightforward to prepare and can be stored in the refrigerator for several days, offering a convenient snack option for busy lifestyles. They also allow for creative flavor combinations to suit individual tastes.

ingredients list:

- 2 cups of quick oats
- 1 cup of shredded coconut
- 3/4 cup of chia seeds
- 1 cup of chocolate chips
- 1/2 cup of honey
- 3/4 cup of creamy peanut butter
- 1/2 teaspoon of vanilla extract

"*Recipe Timeline:*

- **Preparation:** 15 minutes.
- **Cooking:** 12 minutes
- **Total:** 27 minutes"

"To make Chia Seed Energy Balls, follow these steps:

1. Preheat your oven to 350°F (180°C) and line a baking sheet with parchment paper.
2. In a large bowl, mix together oats, coconut, chia seeds, chocolate chips, honey, peanut butter, and vanilla extract until thoroughly combined.
3. Form small portions of the mixture into balls, approximately 2 tablespoons each.
4. Arrange the energy balls on the prepared baking sheet with some space between each one.
5. Bake for 12 minutes, rotating the pan halfway through the baking time.
6. Once baked, allow the energy balls to cool completely on the baking sheet.
7. Transfer the cooled balls to an airtight container for storage.

Energy Bites (per serving, assuming 12-15 energy balls):

- **Energy:** 120-150 calories

Macronutrients:

- **Protein:** 2-3 grams

- **Fat:** 6-8 grams

- **Carbohydrates:** 15-20 grams

- **Fiber:** 3-4 grams

- **Sugar:** 4-6 grams

- **Sodium:** 5-10 milligrams

- **Potassium:** 100-150 milligrams

Vitamins:

- Vitamin A: 10-15% of the Daily Value (DV)
- Vitamin C: 5-10% of the DV
- Calcium: 5-10% of the DV
- Iron: 10-15% of the DV

Other nutrients:

1.Chia seeds: rich in omega-3 fatty acids, protein, and fiber

2.Oats: good source of fiber and beta-glucan

3.Coconut: rich in healthy fats and fiber

4.Chocolate chips: antioxidant-rich and mood-boosting

Please note that this is an estimate and actual values may vary based on the specific ingredients and their measurements used in the recipe.

3. Quinoa Crunch Bars

Quinoa crunch bars are wholesome snack bars primarily made with quinoa, a gluten-free grain known for its high protein and fiber content. Here's a basic rundown of how they're typically prepared:

"Just two ingredients are required to make these tasty treats:"

1. Toasted quinoa (also known as popped quinoa): You can make your own in minutes or use store-bought puffed quinoa. Alternatively, you can substitute with other popped grains like amaranth, rice, or farro.
2. Chocolate chips: Choose your favorite type, such as semi-sweet, dark, milk chocolate, or

Lily's dark chocolate chips for a refined sugar-free option.

Optional: Coconut oil to help melt the chocolate and give it a glossy finish."

"Use a small pan to toast quinoa, enabling you to keep a close eye on the process and prevent burning or over-toasting."

"To pop quinoa:

1. Moisten quinoa with a small amount of water (4:1 ratio).
2. Add a scoop to a medium-high heated pan, flattening it into a single layer.
3. Wait for the water to evaporate and the quinoa to dry out.
4. Break up the quinoa with a whisk as it starts to crackle and pop.
5. Shake the pan to distribute heat evenly.

6. Remove from heat within 15-30 seconds, when the quinoa turns golden brown and emits a toasted, nutty aroma."

"Instructions:

1. Microwave chocolate chips for 60 seconds or use a double boiler to melt them.
2. Combine melted chocolate with popped quinoa until thoroughly mixed.
3. The mixture will become thick and chunky.
4. Line a small glass container or loaf pan (6-7.5 inches) with parchment paper.
5. Pour in the chocolate-quinoa mixture and smooth the surface.
6. Optionally, sprinkle additional popped quinoa on top.
7. Freeze for about 20 minutes until the chocolate sets.
8. Remove the bar from the container using the parchment paper.
9. Allow it to sit at room temperature for a few minutes.

10. Cut into desired portions (e.g., 4 bars or 8 squares).

11. Tip: Run a knife under hot water before slicing for cleaner cuts.

Nutrition Facts:
- per serving:
- Calories: 191
- Macronutrients:
-   Carbohydrates: 29g
-   Protein: 4g
-   Fat: 7g
- Fatty Acid Breakdown:
-   Saturated: 3g
-   Polyunsaturated: 1g
-   Monounsaturated: 0.3g
-   Trans: 0.04g
- Cholesterol: 3mg
- Sodium: 16mg
- Potassium: 120mg
- Fiber: 2g
- Sugar: 14g

- Vitamins and Minerals:
- Vitamin A: 53IU
- Vitamin C: 0.1mg
- Calcium: 36mg
- Iron: 1mg

Explore a variety of snack and treat options! Whether you're seeking nutritious snacks, decadent treats packed with health benefits, or energy bars to power your day, these recipes provide tasty selections for any situation.

Chapter 9: Beverages for Balance

Explore a diverse selection of carefully curated beverages designed to enhance your daily routine. This section delves into crafting drinks that go beyond mere hydration, featuring calming herbal infusions and invigorating smoothies that nourish both body and soul. Discover rejuvenating recipes crafted to support your wellness journey, ensuring each sip contributes to your vitality and overall well-being.

Hydrating Infusions and Teas

Making sure you stay well-hydrated is essential for your overall health. Apart from drinking water, hydrating infusions and teas provide tasty ways to maintain hydration levels and offer extra health advantages:

1. Hydrating Infusions:

These beverages are made by infusing water with fruits, herbs, and occasionally vegetables, offering essential vitamins and minerals. Varieties include cucumber and mint water, citrus-infused water, and berry-infused water.

Sample Recipes

1. Cucumber Mint Water

"Cucumber mint water is a hydrating drink made by infusing water with cucumber slices and fresh mint leaves. It's valued for its subtle flavor and perceived health benefits. Cucumber adds a mild, slightly sweet taste, enhanced by the cooling effect of mint. This blend is popular among those looking to stay hydrated without added sugars or artificial ingredients. To prepare at home, simply combine sliced cucumber and mint leaves with water and let it infuse in the refrigerator for a few hours.

"Beat the heat with this quick and easy Cucumber Mint Water! Ready in just 5 minutes, this refreshing drink is perfect for summer. It's a healthy option with zero calories and no added sugar."

"Stay hydrated with this revitalizing recipe! Water is essential for our bodies, transporting nutrients, oxygen, and flushing out toxins. But we understand plain water can be boring. That's why we have an exciting solution for you! This cucumber mint infused water is simple to make and adds a delightful twist to your hydration routine.

"How much water should you drink daily? Staying hydrated is vital for optimal bodily functions, healthy skin, and mental clarity. It's an easy way to enhance your well-being! Replace sugary beverages with water and notice the difference. Aim to drink half your body weight in ounces of water each day (e.g., 75 ounces if you weigh 150 pounds). This will help keep you hydrated and support overall health."

"Here's what you'll need:

Ingredients:
- Thinly sliced cucumber
- Thinly sliced lime (with peel intact)
- Tightly packed mint leaves
- Water

"Recipe Timeline:
- **Prep time:** 5 minutes.
- **Total time:** 5 minutes."

Instructions:
1. Place cucumber, lime, and mint into a spacious pitcher.
2. Cover the ingredients with water and chill for at least 4 hours, or overnight for the best taste.
3. Savor your revitalizing beverage!

2.Herbal Teas: In addition to keeping you hydrated, herbal teas such as chamomile promote relaxation and aid digestion. Ginger tea is beneficial for alleviating nausea and reducing inflammation. Green tea contains antioxidants and can boost metabolism.

Cucumber mint water is essentially water infused with cucumber slices and mint leaves, containing minimal calories, carbohydrates, protein, fat, and fiber. Cucumbers are mostly water (about 95%), so the nutritional content of cucumber mint water comes mainly from the small amount of carbohydrates and nutrients released by the cucumber and mint. It's a refreshing and hydrating drink with very few calories and insignificant macronutrient content.

9.2 Nutrient-Packed Smoothies and Juices

"Nutrient-packed smoothies and juices" are beverages created by blending or juicing fruits, vegetables, and occasionally nuts, seeds, or yogurt. These drinks are esteemed for their rich nutritional profile, often comprising vitamins, minerals, antioxidants, and fiber. They are favored for their potential health advantages, such as bolstering immune function, enhancing digestion, and offering a convenient means to ingest a diverse array of nutrients in a single serving. Smoothies typically retain the fiber from ingredients, while juices extract the liquid, leaving some fiber behind. Both can be tailored to meet individual preferences and nutritional requirements.

1.Smoothies: Blends of fruits, vegetables, yogurt or milk, and sometimes protein powders or nuts provide fiber, vitamins, and minerals. Green smoothies with spinach or kale offer vitamins A, C, and K.

2.Juices: Freshly squeezed juices deliver concentrated vitamins and minerals. Orange juice is known for vitamin C and beetroot juice for antioxidants and potential blood pressure benefits. Moderation is key due to natural sugars.

9.3 Relaxing Drinks for Evening

"Relaxing drinks for the evening" in the context of vestibular migraine are beverages that can help ease or alleviate symptoms commonly associated with this condition. Vestibular migraines, characterized by vertigo, dizziness, and sensitivity to light and sound, often require lifestyle adjustments, including dietary choices.

Here are examples of calming drinks that may benefit individuals experiencing vestibular migraines in the evening:

1.Herbal Teas: Chamomile, peppermint, and ginger teas are known for their soothing properties. Chamomile, in particular, has traditionally been used to reduce stress and promote relaxation, potentially aiding in managing migraine symptoms.

2. Decaffeinated Green Tea: Green tea contains antioxidants that may have anti-inflammatory effects, which could help reduce migraine symptoms. Choosing decaffeinated varieties avoids potential triggers associated with caffeine.

3.Warm Milk: Milk contains tryptophan, an amino acid that promotes relaxation and may aid in sleep. Adding honey can enhance its soothing effects.

4.Fruit Infused Water: Staying hydrated is crucial for managing migraines. Adding slices of fruits like cucumber, lemon, or berries to water not only enhances flavor but also provides essential nutrients and antioxidants.

5.Golden Milk (Turmeric Milk): Turmeric, known for its anti-inflammatory properties, may help alleviate migraine symptoms. Golden milk, made with turmeric, milk, and honey, can be a comforting drink before bedtime.

6. Cherry Juice: Tart cherry juice has been studied for its potential to reduce inflammation and improve sleep quality, both of which are beneficial for migraine management.

When choosing relaxing drinks, it's important to avoid triggers that could worsen migraine symptoms, such as caffeine, alcohol, or artificial sweeteners. Keeping a diary to track how different beverages affect symptoms can help identify personal triggers and preferences.

Incorporating these calming and hydrating beverages into an evening routine can complement other migraine management strategies, promoting a more restful night's sleep and potentially easing migraine symptoms.

2.Calming beverages can aid relaxation and sleep quality as the day ends:

1.Herbal Infusions:
Herbal infusions, also known as herbal teas or tisanes, have been cherished across diverse cultures for centuries due to their medicinal and therapeutic properties. Unlike traditional teas derived from the Camellia sinensis plant, herbal infusions are crafted from dried leaves, flowers, fruits, seeds, or roots of various herbs and

plants. They are typically caffeine-free and can be enjoyed either hot or cold, depending on personal preference and desired health benefits.

Health Benefits of Herbal Infusions

1.Digestive Health: Herbs like peppermint, chamomile, and ginger aid digestion, alleviate stomach discomfort, and reduce bloating.

2.Relaxation and Stress Relief: Lavender, lemon balm, and passionflower have calming properties that help reduce stress and anxiety, and promote relaxation.

3.Immune Support: Echinacea, elderberry, and ginger boost the immune system, aiding in fighting off colds and flu.

4. Antioxidant Power: Rich in antioxidants, herbal infusions combat free radicals, potentially lowering the risk of chronic diseases.

5. Hydration: Herbal teas contribute to daily fluid intake, promoting overall hydration.

Popular Herbs Used in Herbal Infusions

1. Chamomile: Known for its mild, floral taste and calming effects.

2. Peppermint: Refreshing and widely used for digestive benefits and a cooling sensation.

3. Lavender: Offers a soothing aroma and taste, beneficial for relaxation and stress relief.

4. Ginger: Spicy and warming, supports digestion and immune function.

5.Echinacea: Boosts the immune system, particularly during seasonal illnesses.

6. Hibiscus: Tart and vibrant, rich in antioxidants, and known for its cooling properties.

7.Lemon Balm: Citrusy and calming, enhances mood and relaxation.

How to Prepare Herbal Infusions

1.Basic Preparation:

- Boil water and steep 1-2 teaspoons of dried herbs per cup.

- Cover and steep for 5-10 minutes, adjusting to desired strength.

- Strain and enjoy plain or sweetened with honey, lemon, or other flavors.

2. Cold Infusions:
- Steep herbs in cold water in the refrigerator overnight for a refreshing cold beverage.

3. Herb Combinations:
- Experiment with different herb blends to create unique flavors and enhance health benefits.

Choosing Quality Herbal Infusions

1. Sourcing: Select herbs from reputable suppliers to ensure potency and quality.

2. Organic vs. Conventional: Opt for organic herbs to avoid pesticides and chemicals.

3. Freshness: Choose aromatic, fresh herbs for optimal flavor and benefits.

Herbal infusions provide a delightful way to enjoy the therapeutic benefits of various herbs while supporting overall wellness. Whether seeking relaxation, digestive aid, or immune support, there's an herbal infusion to suit every preference and health need. Through exploring diverse herbs and preparation methods, individuals can uncover a wealth of flavors and health advantages in each cup. Integrate herbal infusions into daily routines for a natural enhancement of well-being.

2. Warm Milk with Spices

Warm milk with spices is a traditional beverage known for its soothing qualities that may provide comfort and potential relief for symptoms associated with vestibular migraine. Vestibular migraine presents with dizziness, vertigo, and other vestibular symptoms, in addition to typical migraine symptoms like headaches and sensitivity to light and sound. While warm milk with spices cannot cure vestibular migraine, certain ingredients in this drink may offer benefits that help in managing symptoms.

Ingredients and Benefits

1. Milk: Milk is rich in calcium and vitamin D, essential for bone health and overall well-being. It is often considered soothing and may help relax muscles and reduce tension.

2. Spices: Various spices are added for flavor and potential health benefits, including:

1.Turmeric is known for its anti-inflammatory properties, which may help reduce inflammation associated with migraines.

2.Cinnamon: Contains antioxidants and may aid in regulating blood sugar levels.

2.Ginger: Well-known for its anti-nausea properties, ginger may alleviate nausea linked to migraines.

3.Cardamom: Offers digestive benefits and enhances the drink's flavor.

4.Nutmeg: Adds a calming aroma and flavor to the beverage.

Potential Benefits for Vestibular Migraine

While scientific evidence linking warm milk with spices directly to treating vestibular migraine is limited, the components in this beverage may provide potential benefits:

1.Relaxation: Warm milk is commonly believed to promote relaxation and reduce stress, potentially beneficial during a migraine attack.

2. Anti-inflammatory Effects: Ingredients such as turmeric and ginger possess anti-inflammatory properties that could help alleviate migraine-related inflammation.

3. Nausea Relief: Ginger, in particular, is effective in reducing nausea, a common symptom in vestibular migraine.

4. Hydration: Milk provides hydration, essential during migraine episodes to prevent dehydration, which can trigger migraines.

To prepare warm milk with spices:

1. Heat one cup of milk (dairy or non-dairy) in a saucepan until warm but not boiling.

2. Add a pinch of turmeric, cinnamon, ginger, cardamom, and nutmeg to the milk, adjusting to taste.

3. Stir well and allow the flavors to meld for a few minutes.

4. Optionally, sweeten with honey or another sweetener as desired.

5. Consume slowly while warm for optimal effect.

Warm milk with spices offers a comforting option that may provide relief and comfort during episodes of vestibular migraine. While individual responses may vary, the combination of milk, turmeric, ginger, and other spices presents potential benefits such as anti-inflammatory effects, nausea relief, and overall relaxation. It can complement medical treatments and lifestyle adjustments as part of a holistic approach to managing vestibular migraine symptoms. For personalized advice and treatment options, always consult a healthcare professional.

3. Golden Milk

Golden Milk, also known as turmeric milk or turmeric latte, is a traditional Indian beverage renowned for its health benefits, primarily due to its main ingredient, turmeric. Turmeric contains curcumin, known for its anti-inflammatory and antioxidant properties. Vestibular migraine is a neurological condition characterized by vertigo and dizziness, and often accompanied by migraine headaches. While treatment usually involves medications and lifestyle adjustments, some individuals explore complementary therapies like Golden Milk for symptom relief and management.

Turmeric and Curcumin: Key Components of Golden Milk

1.Curcumin: Found in turmeric, curcumin has potential health benefits, particularly its anti-inflammatory effects, which may help reduce inflammation in the nervous system and alleviate symptoms of vestibular migraines.

2.Anti-inflammatory Properties: Inflammation is believed to contribute to migraines, including vestibular migraines. Curcumin's anti-inflammatory properties may help alleviate symptoms such as vertigo and dizziness during migraine attacks.

Benefits of Golden Milk for Vestibular Migraine

1.Anti-inflammatory Effects: Curcumin's anti-inflammatory properties may provide relief from symptoms experienced during vestibular migraine attacks.

2.Antioxidant Properties: Turmeric's antioxidants can neutralize free radicals, potentially reducing oxidative stress associated with migraine attacks.

3.Neuroprotective Effects: Some studies suggest curcumin may have neuroprotective effects, beneficial for managing the neurological symptoms of vestibular migraine.

Incorporating Golden Milk into Your Routine

2.Preparation: Golden Milk is typically made by heating milk (dairy or non-dairy) with turmeric and spices like black pepper, cinnamon, and ginger, not only enhancing flavor but also offering additional health benefits.

2.Frequency and Considerations: Before adding Golden Milk to your routine, especially if you're on medications or have health concerns, consult with a healthcare provider to ensure it's safe and suitable for you.

Considerations and Precautions

2.Medication Interactions: Curcumin may interact with certain medications, such as blood thinners. Consult a healthcare provider to determine if Golden Milk is appropriate for your health condition.

3.Individual Responses: Responses to Golden Milk may vary; some individuals may find relief from symptoms, while others may not experience significant benefits.

Conclusion

Golden Milk, enriched with turmeric and curcumin, offers potential as a complementary approach to managing symptoms of vestibular migraine due to its anti-inflammatory and antioxidant properties. While more research specific to vestibular migraine is needed, its potential benefits warrant consideration alongside medical treatment and consultation with healthcare providers to ensure comprehensive migraine management.

Choosing beverages that maintain hydration, provide nutrients, and promote relaxation is integral to overall well-being. Incorporating hydrating infusions, nutrient-packed smoothies and juices, and calming evening drinks into daily routines supports a balanced and healthy lifestyle.

This chapter aims to guide readers in selecting beverages that contribute positively to health and relaxation goals while ensuring hydration and nutrient intake.

Chapter 10: Meal Planning and Preparation Tips

Chapter 10 offers an extensive manual on mastering meal planning and preparation. It covers effective grocery shopping methods and time-saving cooking techniques, providing essential skills to simplify your culinary routine. Discover how to craft well-balanced menus, creatively use leftovers, and leverage batch cooking to manage hectic schedules. Whether you're new to cooking or an experienced chef, these insights are designed to enhance kitchen efficiency and ensure you savor delicious, nutritious meals daily.

Creating Weekly Meal Plans

Structured meal planning can significantly aid those with vestibular migraine in managing symptoms by ensuring balanced meals and avoiding triggers. Key steps include:

1.Identifying Trigger Foods: Consult with a healthcare provider to pinpoint common triggers like aged cheeses, caffeine, or processed meats.

2.Balancing Macronutrients: Aim for meals with a mix of carbohydrates, proteins, and healthy fats to stabilize blood sugar and support overall health.

3.Incorporating Anti-Inflammatory Foods: Include omega-3-rich foods (e.g., salmon, flaxseeds) and antioxidants (e.g., berries, leafy greens) to reduce inflammation linked to migraines.

4.Planning Regular, Small Meals: Consistent eating times and smaller portions throughout the day can prevent hunger-induced migraines.

Tips for Grocery Shopping

Efficient grocery shopping is crucial for maintaining a migraine-friendly diet:

1.Creating a List: Plan meals and make a detailed shopping list to avoid impulse buys and ensure you have all the necessary ingredients.

2.Shopping the Perimeter: Focus on fresh produce, lean proteins, and dairy found around the store's edges, as these are typically less processed.

3.Checking Labels: Read ingredient lists carefully for potential triggers such as additives, preservatives, and high sodium or sugar content.

4.Considering Online Shopping: Online options can reduce sensory triggers like bright lights and strong odors often found in physical stores.

10.3 Batch Cooking and Freezing Meals

Preparing meals in advance can save time and energy during migraine attacks:

2.Choosing Migraine-Safe Recipes:
Cook large batches of soups, stews, or casseroles using fresh ingredients and migraine-friendly seasonings.

3.Using Proper Storage:
Store meals in BPA-free containers or freezer bags, clearly labeled with continents and date for easy reheating.

4.Freezer-Friendly Options:
Freeze portions of cooked grains, proteins, and vegetables to quickly assemble balanced meals.

Following these tailored meal planning and preparation strategies can assist individuals with vestibular migraine in managing symptoms and promoting overall well-being through a nutritious diet. Always consult with healthcare professionals for personalized guidance and to identify specific triggers unique to your health condition.

Chapter 11: Lifestyle Strategies for Managing Vestibular Migraines

Chapter 11 of "Lifestyle Strategies for Managing Vestibular Migraines" focuses on practical methods individuals can use to reduce symptoms and enhance their quality of life. It begins by addressing the unique challenges of vestibular migraines, such as dizziness, vertigo, and sensitivity to light and sound, stressing the need for a comprehensive approach that combines medical treatments with lifestyle changes.

The chapter offers a detailed exploration of lifestyle adjustments that can significantly reduce symptoms. These include dietary changes, stress management techniques, improving sleep hygiene, and tailored exercise routines designed for those experiencing vestibular migraine symptoms. Each of these factors is highlighted for its role in influencing the frequency and severity of migraines.

Moreover, the chapter discusses the importance of identifying and avoiding triggers, providing practical advice on creating environments at home and work that minimize migraine triggers.

Additionally, the benefits of mindfulness and relaxation techniques in reducing stress, a common trigger for migraines, are explored in depth. The chapter provides specific guidance on incorporating practices like meditation and deep breathing exercises into daily routines.

Overall, Chapter 11 serves as a practical handbook, equipping readers with knowledge and strategies to actively manage vestibular migraines through lifestyle adjustments. It emphasizes the need for a personalized approach, encouraging individuals to experiment with different techniques to find what best suits their health and symptom management goals.

Stress Management Techniques

Stress is a significant trigger for vestibular migraines. Implementing effective stress management techniques can reduce the frequency and severity of attacks. Here are some strategies:

1.Mindfulness and Meditation: Practicing mindfulness and meditation helps regulate stress levels by promoting relaxation and reducing anxiety.

2.Deep Breathing Exercises: Techniques like diaphragmatic breathing calm the nervous system and alleviate stress.

3.Progressive Muscle Relaxation: This method involves tensing and then relaxing muscle groups to promote physical and mental relaxation.

4.Cognitive Behavioral Therapy (CBT): CBT techniques help identify and change negative thought patterns and behaviors contributing to stress.

5.Time Management: Organizing tasks and setting priorities reduces stress by providing a sense of control.

Importance of Regular Exercise

Regular physical activity not only improves overall health but also helps manage vestibular migraines:

1.Cardiovascular Exercise: Activities such as walking, jogging, swimming, or cycling improve blood flow and reduce migraine frequency.

2. Strength Training: Building muscle enhances fitness and resilience to stress, potentially reducing migraine triggers.

3. Yoga and Stretching: These practices improve flexibility, reduce muscle tension, and promote relaxation, aiding in migraine management.

4. Consistency: Establishing a regular exercise routine is crucial. Aim for at least 30 minutes of moderate exercise most days of the week.

Sleep Hygiene Practices

Quality sleep is essential for managing vestibular migraines and overall well-being. Adopting good sleep hygiene practices can enhance sleep quality:

1. Consistent Sleep Schedule: Going to bed and waking up at the same time daily regulates your body's internal clock.

2. Create a Relaxing Bedtime Routine: Engage in calming activities before bed, such as reading or taking a warm bath, to signal relaxation.

3. Optimize Your Sleep Environment: Ensure your bedroom is cool, quiet, and dark. Use comfortable bedding and consider blackout curtains or a white noise machine if needed.

4. Limit Stimulants and Screen Time: Avoid caffeine and electronics before bed as they can disrupt sleep.

5. Manage Stress and Anxiety: Techniques like meditation or journaling before bed can clear your mind and promote relaxation.

By integrating these lifestyle strategies into your daily routine, you can better manage vestibular migraines and improve your overall quality of life. Collaborate with healthcare providers to tailor these strategies to your individual needs and health goals.

Extra Bonus : 30-Day Meal Prep Plan"

This 30-day meal prep plan incorporates a variety of nutritious meals designed to potentially support individuals managing vestibular migraines. Each day offers balanced options focusing on whole grains, lean proteins, healthy fats, and plenty of fruits and vegetables. Adjust portion sizes and ingredients as needed based on individual preferences and dietary requirements.

Week 1:

- **Day 1- Breakfast:** Overnight oats with mixed berries

- **Lunch:** Grilled chicken salad with mixed greens, cucumber, and balsamic vinaigrette

- **_Dinner:_** Baked salmon with roasted sweet potatoes and steamed broccoli

- **_Day 2- Breakfast:_** Greek yogurt with honey and almonds

- **_Lunch:_** Quinoa and black bean stuffed bell peppers

- **_Dinner:_** Turkey meatballs with whole wheat pasta and marinara sauce

- **_Day 3 Breakfast:_** Smoothie with spinach, banana, and almond milk

- **_Lunch:_** Lentil soup with whole grain bread

- **_Dinner:_** Grilled shrimp skewers with quinoa salad

- **_Day 4 Breakfast:_** Chia seed pudding with mango and coconut flakes

- **_Lunch:_** Spinach and avocado salad with grilled chicken

- **_Dinner:_** Baked cod with quinoa and roasted vegetables

- **_Day 5-Breakfast:_** Whole grain toast with almond butter and sliced banana

- **_Lunch:_** Tuna salad wrap with whole wheat tortilla

- **_Dinner:_** Stir-fried tofu with brown rice and mixed vegetables

Week 2:

- **_Day 6- Breakfast:_** Cottage cheese with pineapple and walnuts

- **_Lunch:_** Mediterranean chickpea salad

- **_Dinner:_** Baked chicken breast with sweet potato fries and green beans

- **_Day 7- Breakfast:_** Whole grain pancakes with berries and a drizzle of honey

- **_Lunch:_** Caprese salad with mozzarella, tomatoes, and basil

- **_Dinner:_** Beef stir-fry with broccoli and brown rice

- **_Day 8 - Breakfast:_** Oatmeal with diced apples and cinnamon

- **_Lunch:_** Chicken Caesar salad with whole grain croutons

- **_Dinner:_** Grilled swordfish with quinoa and asparagus

- **_Day 9- Breakfast_:** Yogurt parfait with granola and mixed berries

- **_Lunch:_** Lentil and vegetable stew

- **_Dinner:_** Turkey burgers with whole wheat buns and side salad

- **_Day 10- Breakfast:_** Smoothie bowl with kiwi, strawberries, and granola

- **_Lunch:_** Quinoa tabbouleh with cucumber and mint

- **_Dinner:_** Baked tofu with stir-fried vegetables and brown rice

Week 3:

- **_Day 11- Breakfast_:** Scrambled eggs with spinach and whole grain toast

- **Lunch:** Spinach and feta stuffed portobello mushrooms

- **Dinner:** Salmon filet with quinoa pilaf and roasted Brussels sprouts

- **Day 12 - Breakfast:** Banana and almond butter smoothie

- **Lunch:** Greek salad with grilled chicken

- **Dinner**: Turkey chili with cornbread muffins

- **Day 13 - Breakfast:** Acai bowl with granola, coconut flakes, and berries

- **Lunch:** Vegetable stir-fry with tofu and brown rice

- **Dinner:** Baked halibut with quinoa and steamed vegetables

- **_Day 14 - Breakfast:_** Whole grain waffles with yogurt and mixed fruit

- **_Lunch:_** Chickpea and kale salad with lemon tahini dressing

- **_Dinner:_** Grilled chicken thighs with sweet potato mash and green beans

- **_Day 15 - Breakfast:_** Overnight chia seed pudding with raspberries and honey

- **_Lunch:_** Quinoa stuffed zucchini boats

- **_Dinner:_** Beef and broccoli stir-fry with brown rice

Week 4:

- **_Day 16 - Breakfast:_** Smoothie with mango, pineapple, and coconut water

- **_Lunch:_** Mediterranean tuna salad with mixed greens

- **_Dinner:_** Baked cod with quinoa and roasted vegetables

- **_Day 17 - Breakfast:_** Whole grain toast with avocado and poached eggs

- **_Lunch:_** Lentil soup with whole grain bread

- **_Dinner:_** Chicken fajitas with whole wheat tortillas and guacamole

- **_Day 18 - Breakfast:_** Greek yogurt with honey, almonds, and fresh berries

- **_Lunch:_** Caprese quinoa salad

- **_Dinner:_** Stir-fried shrimp with vegetables and brown rice

- **_Day 19 - Breakfast:_** Oatmeal with sliced banana and walnuts

- **_Lunch:_** Spinach and chickpea salad with lemon vinaigrette

- **_Dinner:_** Turkey meatballs with marinara sauce over spaghetti squash

- **_Day 20- Breakfast:_** Smoothie bowl with spinach, berries, and almond butter

- **_Lunch:_** Quinoa and black bean burrito bowl

- **_Dinner_**: Grilled salmon with quinoa tabbouleh and steamed asparagus

Week 5:

- ***Day 21- Breakfast:*** Greek yogurt with berries and a sprinkle of almonds.

- ***Lunch:*** Quinoa salad with spinach, cherry tomatoes, and grilled chicken.

- ***Dinner:*** Baked salmon with steamed asparagus and brown rice.

- ***Day 22- Breakfast:*** Smoothie with spinach, banana, almond milk, and chia seeds.

- ***Lunch:*** Lentil soup with a side of mixed greens salad.

- ***Dinner:*** Turkey meatballs with zucchini noodles and marinara sauce.

- ***Day 23- Breakfast:*** Oatmeal topped with sliced apples and a drizzle of honey.

- **Lunch:** Grilled shrimp with quinoa and roasted vegetables.

- **Dinner:** Stir-fried tofu with broccoli and bell peppers over brown rice.

- **Day 24- Breakfast:** Whole grain toast with avocado spread and poached eggs.

- **Lunch:** Chicken and vegetable stir-fry with brown rice.

- **Dinner:** Baked cod with roasted sweet potatoes and green beans.

- **Day 25- Breakfast:** Cottage cheese with sliced peaches and a sprinkle of sunflower seeds.

- **Lunch:** Spinach salad with grilled steak slices and balsamic vinaigrette.

- **_Dinner:_** Stuffed bell peppers with ground turkey, quinoa, and tomato sauce.

- **_Day 26- Breakfast:_** Smoothie bowl with mixed berries, almond milk, and granola.

- **_Lunch:_** Whole wheat wrap with hummus, grilled chicken, and mixed greens.

- **_Dinner:_** Baked chicken breast with steamed broccoli and wild rice.

- **_Day 27-Breakfast:_** Scrambled eggs with spinach and feta cheese.

- **_Lunch:_** Lentil and vegetable stew.

- **_Dinner:_** Grilled salmon with quinoa and sautéed kale.

- **_Day 28- Breakfast:_** Yogurt parfait with granola and sliced strawberries.

- **Lunch:** Turkey and avocado whole wheat sandwich with a side salad.

- **Dinner:** Beef and vegetable kebabs with couscous.

- **Day 29- Breakfast:** Chia seed pudding with almond milk and fresh fruit.

- **Lunch:** Quinoa and black bean salad with grilled shrimp.

- **Dinner:** Baked tilapia with roasted Brussels sprouts and sweet potato mash.

- **Day 30- Breakfast:** Whole grain pancakes with maple syrup and a side of mixed fruit.

- **Lunch:** Chicken Caesar salad with whole wheat croutons.

- ***Dinner:*** Vegetarian chili with a side of cornbread.

This meal plan emphasizes healthy, well-rounded meals tailored for those on a vestibular migraine diet. Each day features a mix of proteins, whole grains, fruits, and vegetables to provide a balanced and enjoyable eating regimen. Adjust serving sizes and ingredients as per personal dietary requirements and tastes.

Embracing a Balanced Lifestyle with Vestibular Migraines

Living with vestibular migraines necessitates a holistic strategy to manage symptoms and maintain overall well-being. These migraines, a neurological condition, manifest with vertigo, dizziness, and other vestibular symptoms, often accompanied by typical migraine indicators such as headaches, sensitivity to light and sound, and nausea. Effective management involves medical treatment, lifestyle adjustments, and self-care strategies aimed at reducing the frequency and severity of attacks while improving quality of life.

Medical Management

1. Consultation and Diagnosis: Accurate diagnosis by a neurologist or migraine specialist is crucial for effective treatment planning.

2. Medication: Treatment may include preventive medications to reduce migraine frequency or abortive medications to alleviate symptoms during attacks. Over-the-counter pain relievers may also be recommended.

3. Therapies: Physical therapy, vestibular rehabilitation, and cognitive-behavioral therapy (CBT) can help manage symptoms, improve balance, and address the emotional impact of chronic migraines.

Lifestyle Adjustments

1. Identifying Triggers: Keeping a migraine diary helps identify triggers like stress, certain foods, hormonal changes, or environmental factors to minimize exposure.

2. Sleep Hygiene: Establishing a regular sleep schedule and creating a conducive sleep environment can reduce migraines triggered by sleep disturbances.

3. Dietary Modifications: Avoiding trigger foods such as caffeine, alcohol, and processed foods, while maintaining a balanced diet rich in fruits, vegetables, and whole grains, supports overall health and reduces migraine frequency.

4. Hydration: Staying hydrated is crucial as dehydration can trigger migraines in some individuals.

5. Stress Management: Incorporating stress-reduction techniques like mindfulness meditation, yoga, deep breathing exercises, or engaging in hobbies can effectively manage stress, a common migraine trigger.

Self-Care Strategies

1. Regular Exercise: Engaging in activities such as walking, swimming, or cycling can reduce migraine severity and frequency, promoting overall physical and mental well-being.

2. Work-Life Balance: Balancing work, personal life, and rest is essential. Avoiding overexertion and taking regular breaks during activities can help prevent migraines.

3. Support Network: Building a supportive network of friends, family, or support groups provides emotional support and practical assistance during migraine episodes.

Conclusion

Embracing a balanced lifestyle with vestibular migraines involves integrating medical management, lifestyle adjustments, and self-care strategies. Collaboration with healthcare professionals, identifying triggers, making necessary lifestyle changes, and implementing effective self-care practices can significantly reduce the impact of vestibular migraines and enhance overall quality of life. Regular monitoring and adjustments to the treatment plan are vital for optimal management and continued well-being.

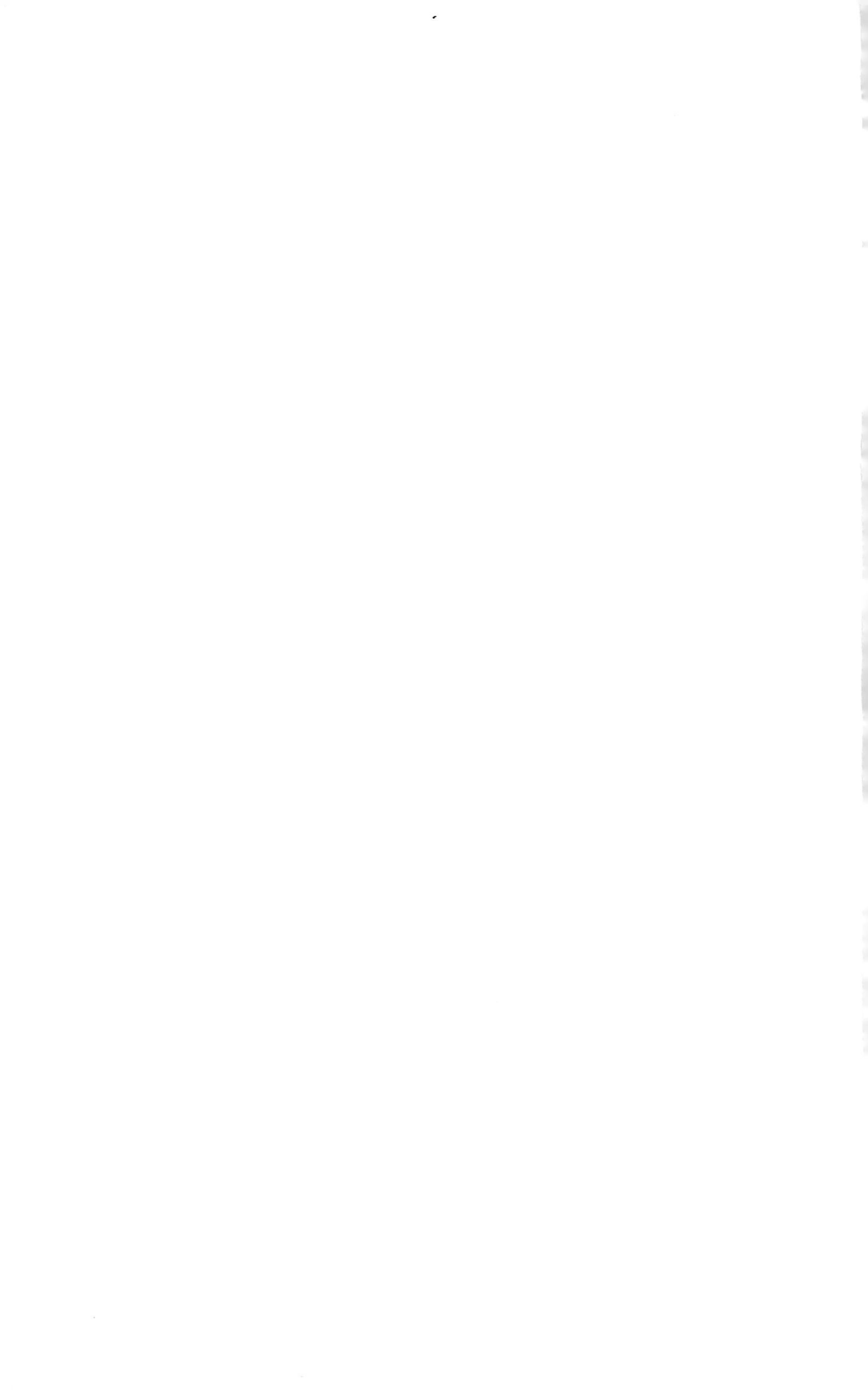

Made in United States
Troutdale, OR
04/28/2025